50 Studies Every Obstetrician-Gynecologist
Should Know

50 STUDIES EVERY DOCTOR SHOULD KNOW

50 Studies Every Doctor Should Know: The Key Studies that Form the Foundation of Evidence Based Medicine, Revised Edition
Michael E. Hochman

50 Studies Every Internist Should Know
Kristopher Swiger, Joshua R. Thomas, Michael E. Hochman, and Steven Hochman

50 Studies Every Neurologist Should Know
David Y. Hwang and David M. Greer

50 Studies Every Pediatrician Should Know
Ashaunta T. Anderson, Nina L. Shapiro, Stephen C. Aronoff, Jeremiah Davis, and Michael Levy

50 Imaging Studies Every Doctor Should Know
Christoph I. Lee

50 Studies Every Surgeon Should Know
SreyRam Kuy, Rachel J. Kwon, and Miguel A. Burch

50 Studies Every Intensivist Should Know
Edward A. Bittner

50 Studies Every Palliative Care Doctor Should Know
David Hui, Akhila Reddy, and Eduardo Bruera

50 Studies Every Psychiatrist Should Know
Ish P. Bhalla, Rajesh R. Tampi, and Vinod H. Srihari

50 Studies Every Anesthesiologist Should Know
Anita Gupta, Michael E. Hochman, Elena N. Gutman

50 Studies Every Ophthalmologist Should Know
Alan D. Penman, Kimberly W. Crowder, and William M. Watkins, Jr.

50 Studies Every Urologist Should Know
Philipp Dahm

50 Studies Every Obstetrician-Gynecologist Should Know
Constance Liu, Noah Rindos, and Scott A. Shainker

50 Studies Every Obstetrician-Gynecologist Should Know

EDITED BY

Constance Liu, MD, PhD
Medical Offficer
Department of Obstetrics and Gynecology
Gallup Indian Medical Center
Gallup, NM, USA

Noah Rindos, MD
Assistant Professor
Department of Obstetrics and Gynecology
UPMC Magee-Womens Hospital
Pittsburgh, PA, USA

Scott A. Shainker, DO, MS
The Annie and Chase Koch Chair in Obstetrics and Gynecology,
Director, New England Center for Placental Disorder, Assistant Professor
of Obstetrics, Gynecology, and Reproductive Biology
Division of Maternal-Fetal Medicine, Department of Obstetrics
and Gynecology
Beth Israel Deaconess Medical Center/Harvard Medical School
Boston, MA, USA

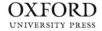

OXFORD
UNIVERSITY PRESS

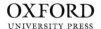

OXFORD
UNIVERSITY PRESS

Oxford University Press is a department of the University of Oxford. It furthers
the University's objective of excellence in research, scholarship, and education
by publishing worldwide. Oxford is a registered trade mark of Oxford University
Press in the UK and certain other countries.

Published in the United States of America by Oxford University Press
198 Madison Avenue, New York, NY 10016, United States of America.

Library of Congress Cataloging-in-Publication Data
Names: Liu, Constance, editor. | Rindos, Noah, editor. | Shainker A., Scott, editor.
Title: 50 studies every obstetrician-gynecologist should know /
[edited by] Constance Liu, Noah Rindos, Scott A. Shainker.
Other titles: Fifty studies every obstetrician and gynecologist should know |
50 studies every doctor should know (Series)
Description: New York, NY : Oxford University Press, 2021. |
Series: 50 studies every doctor should know |
Includes bibliographical references and index.
Identifiers: LCCN 2020036319 (print) | LCCN 2020036320 (ebook) | ISBN 9780190947088 (paperback) |
ISBN 9780190947101 (epub) | ISBN 9780190947118 (online)
Subjects: MESH: Pregnancy Complications | Pregnancy | Genital Diseases, Female | Case Reports
Classification: LCC RG525 (print) | LCC RG525 (ebook) | NLM WQ 240 | DDC 618.2—dc23
LC record available at https://lccn.loc.gov/2020036319
LC ebook record available at https://lccn.loc.gov/2020036320

DOI: 10.1093/med/9780190947088.001.0001

To Chris, Taro, and Hiro: I love you like a zebra loves its stripes. Thanks & love to my parents: Drs. Wen-Shin and Wan-tzu.

—Constance Liu

Thank you to Steph, Raspberry, Luca, and Milo for all of your support and love.

—Noah Rindos

To Mom, Lindsay, Molly, and Logan for their unending love and support.
To my father, who would have received such enjoyment from this . . .

—Scott A. Shainker

CONTENTS

PREFACE FROM THE SERIES EDITOR

When I was a third-year medical student, I asked one of my senior residents—who seemed to be able to quote every medical study in the history of mankind—if he had a list of key studies that have defined the current practice of general medicine that I should read before graduating medical school. "Don't worry," he told me. "You will learn the key studies as you go along."

But picking up on these key studies didn't prove so easy, and I was frequently admonished by my attendings for being unaware of crucial literature in their field. More important, because I had a mediocre understanding of the medical literature at that time, I lacked confidence in my clinical decision-making and had difficulty appreciating the significance of new research findings. It wasn't until I was well into my residency—thanks to considerable amount of effort and determination—that I finally began to feel comfortable with both the emerging and fundamental medical literature.

Now, as a practicing general internist, I realize that I am not the only doctor who has struggled to become familiar with the key medical studies that form the foundation of evidence-based practice. Many of the students and residents I work with tell me that they feel overwhelmed by the medical literature and that they cannot process new research findings because they lack a solid understanding of what has already been published. Even many practicing physicians—including those with years of experience—have only a cursory knowledge of the medical evidence base and make clinical decisions largely on personal experience.

I initially wrote *50 Studies Every Doctor Should Know* in an attempt to provide medical professionals (and even lay readers interested in learning more about medical research) a quick way to get up to speed on the classic studies that shape clinical practice. But it soon became clear there was a greater need for this distillation of the medical evidence than my original book provided. Soon after the book's publication, I began receiving calls from specialist physicians in a variety of disciplines wondering about the possibility of another book focusing on studies in their field. In partnership with a wonderful team of editors from Oxford University Press, we have developed my initial book into a series, offering volumes in Internal Medicine, Pediatrics, Surgery, Neurology, Radiology, Critical Care, Anesthesia, Psychiatry, Palliative Care, Ophthalmology, and now Obstetrics and Gynecology. Several additional volumes are in the works.

I am particularly excited about this latest volume in Obstetrics and Gynecology, which is the culmination of hard work by a team of editors—Constance Liu, Noah Rindos, and Scott A. Shainker, who have summarized the most important studies in their field. Particularly over the past several years, there has become a solid evidence base in the field of Obstetrics and Gynecology, and Drs. Liu, Rindos, and Shainker have effectively captured it in this volume. I believe *50 Studies Every Obstetrician-Gynecologist Should Know* provides the perfect launching ground for trainees in the field as well as a helpful refresher for practicing clinicians–physicians, nurse practitioners, and other women's health professionals. The book also highlights key knowledge gaps that may stimulate researchers to tackle key unanswered questions in the field. A special thanks also goes to the wonderful editors at Oxford University Press—Marta Moldvai and Tiffany Lu—who injected energy and creativity into the production process for this volume. This volume was a pleasure to help develop, and I learned a lot about the field of Obstetrics and Gynecology in the process.

I have no doubt you will gain important insights into the field of Obstetrics and Gynecology in the pages ahead!

Michael E. Hochman, MD, MPH

PREFACE

We entered the field of obstetrics and gynecology eager to learn, advocate for patients, and become the physician-scientists we are today. We believe in reproductive rights and evidence-based medicine: together these foster the ability to provide compassionate and optimal care. We embarked on this project because we believe that understanding the primary literature is critical for any clinician who seeks to practice thoughtful, evidence-based medicine. More than just knowing what to do, we believe clinicians should know why they do it.

This volume, part of the larger series *50 Studies Every Doctor Should Know*, aims to present a foundational understanding of the practice of obstetrics and gynecology. We interrogated a broad range of literature. While there are certainly far more than 50 studies we could have included, we employed a rigorous iterative process that prioritized studies that impact current practice and, importantly, answer the "why" of management. This book is ideal for generalists who seek to contextualize new evidence, practitioners of women's health who wish to deepen their understanding of the literature, trainees who are learning the basics of management, and even the interested lay person who wants to understand what studies are guiding their care.

We are grateful for the contributions of the chapter authors across a diverse range of subspecialties. We thank them for their clinical experience, knowledge, and ability to make these studies accessible to readers at all levels of experience.

Collectively we represent the diverse field of obstetrics and gynecology: (CL) a generalist obstetrician-gynecologist serving Native American patients in rural western New Mexico, (SS) an academic maternal-fetal medicine specialist in Boston, and (NR) a minimally invasive pelvic surgeon in Pittsburgh. From residency at Boston Medical Center, our paths have diverged neatly to represent a range of career choices, but we have this in common: a commitment to advocating for our patients and an understanding that offering the best care means continual attention to our foundation of evidentiary learning. We hope this volume provides additional background for you to achieve the same.

We would like to thank Dr. Michael Hochman for his vision in creating this series. We are also grateful to Ms. Marta Moldvai and Ms. Tiffany Lu from Oxford University Press for their editorial support and guidance. We appreciate the contributions of Justin Dietrich to the family planning section. Finally, we would like to thank the patients who participated in these clinical trials and studies.

Constance Liu, MD, PhD
Noah Rindos, MD
Scott A. Shainker, DO, MS

CONTRIBUTORS

Jodi F. Abbott, MD, MHCM
Associate Professor
Department of Obstetrics and
  Gynecology
Boston University School of Medicine
Boston, MA, USA

Arnold P. Advincula, MD
Professor & Division Chief
Division of Gynecologic Specialty
  Surgery
Columbia University Medical Center
New York, NY, USA

C. Sola Ajewole, MD
Resident Physician
Department of Obstetrics and
  Gynecology
Boston Medical Center
Boston, MA, USA

Chetna Arora, MD
Assistant Professor
Department of Obstetrics and
  Gynecology
Columbia University
New York, NY, USA

Ashley N. Battarbee, MD, MSCR
Assistant Professor
Department of Obstetrics and
  Gynecology
University of Alabama
Birmingham, AL, USA

**Alexandra Belcher-Obejero-Paz,
MD, MPH**
Obstetrics and Gynecology Generalist
Department of Obstetrics and
  Gynecology
Lynn Community Health Center
Lynn, MA, USA

Ashley E. Benson, MD, MA
Physician Fellow
Department of Obstetrics and
  Gynecology
University of Utah
Salt Lake City, UT, USA

Rachel Beverley, MD
Fellow, Reproductive Endocrinology
  and Infertility
Department of Obstetrics,
  Gynecology, and Reproductive
  Sciences
University of Pittsburgh
  Medical Center
Pittsburgh, PA, USA

Rachel Blake, MD
Chief Resident, PGY4
Department of Obstetrics and
  Gynecology
Harvard Medical School
Boston, MA, USA

Megan Bradley, MD
Department of Obstetrics and
  Gynecology
UPMC Magee-Womens Hospital
Pittsburgh, PA, USA

Linda Burkett, MD
Physician, Urogynecology
Department of Obstetrics,
  Gynecology, and REI
UPMC Magee-Womens
  Hospital
Pittsburgh, PA, USA

Chelsea Chandler, MD
Fellow
Department of Gynecologic
  Oncology
UPMC Magee-Womens Hospital
Pittsburgh, PA, USA

Sujata Chouinard, MD
Resident Physician
Department of Obstetrics and
  Gynecology
University of New Mexico
Albuquerque, NM, USA

Sarah L. Cohen, MD, MPH
Minimally Invasive Gynecologic
  Surgeon
Department of Gynecology
Mayo Clinic
Rochester, MN, USA

Zachary Colvin, DO
Maternal Fetal Medicine Fellow
Department of Obstetrics and
  Gynecology
Medical College of Wisconsin
Milwaukee, WI, USA

Antoinette Danvers, MD, MSCR
Assistant Professor
Department of Obstetrics and
  Gynecology and Women's
  Health
Albert Einstein College of Medicine/
  Montefiore Medical Center
Bronx, NY, USA

Shad Deering, MD
Associate Dean, Baylor College of
  Medicine, Children's Hospital
  of San Antonio System Medical
  Director, CHRISTUS Simulation
  Institute
Department of Obstetrics and
  Gynecology
Baylor College of Medicine
Houston, TX, USA

Nicole Donnellan, MD
Associate Professor
Department of Obstetrics,
  Gynecology, and Reproductive
  Sciences
UPMC Magee-Womens Hospital
Pittsburgh, PA, USA

Stephanie Dukhovny, MD
Assistant Professor
Department of Obstetrics and
  Gynecology
OHSU
Portland, OR, USA

Hugh Ehrenberg, MD
Attending Physician
Department of Maternal Fetal
    Medicine
Voorhees, NJ, USA

Brett D. Einerson, MD, MPH
Assistant Professor
Department of Obstetrics and
    Gynecology
University of Utah
Salt Lake City, UT, USA

Hadi Erfani, MD, MPH
Resident
Department of Obstetrics and
    Gynecology
Baylor College of Medicine
Houston, TX, USA

Eve Espey, MD, MPH
Professor and Chair
Department of Obstetrics and
    Gynecology
University of New Mexico
Albuquerque, NM, USA

Mary Louise Fowler, MD, MEng
Resident Physician
Department of Obstetrics and
    Gynecology
Boston Medical Center
Boston, MA, USA

Karin Fox, MD, MEd
Department of Obstetrics and
    Gynecology
Baylor College of Medicine
Houston, TX, USA

Alexis Gadson, MD
REI Fellow
Women and Infants Hospital/Brown
    University
Providence, RI, USA

Alison A. Garrett, MD
Fellow
Department of Gynecologic
    Oncology
UPMC Magee-Womens Hospital
Pittsburgh, PA, USA

Dena Goffman, MD
Chief of Obstetrics
Department of Obstetrics and
    Gynecology
Columbia University Irving
    Medical Center
New York, NY, USA

Toni Golen, MD
Assistant Professor
Department of Obstetrics,
    Gynecology, and Reproductive
    Biology
Beth Israel Deaconess Medical
    Center/Harvard Medical School
Boston, MA, USA

Jaclyn Grentzer, MD, MSCI
Independent Provider
Planned Parenthood of Orange and
    San Bernardino Counties
Laguna Beach, CA, USA

Sadia Haider, MD, MPH
Associate Professor of Obstetrics and
    Gynecology
Department of Obstetrics and
    Gynecology
University of Chicago
Chicago, IL, USA

Jessica M. Hart, MD
Fellow
Department of Maternal Fetal
    Medicine
Beth Israel Deaconess Medical Center
Boston, MA, USA

Christine Helou, MD
Department of Obstetrics and
    Gynecology
Greater Baltimore Medical Center
Towson, MD, USA

Paul Hendessi, MD
Clinical Associate Professor
Department of Obstetrics and
    Gynecology
Boston University
Boston, MA, USA

Jonathan S. Hirshberg, MD
Clinical Fellow in Maternal-Fetal
    Medicine and Surgical Critical Care
Department of Obstetrics and
    Gynecology/Department of
    Surgery
Washington University
St. Louis, MO, USA

Michael Hochman, MD, MPH
Director of the USC Gehr Family
    Center for Health Systems
    Science and Innovation
Internal Medicine
Keck School of Medicine of USC
Sherman, Oaks, CA

Michael House, MD
Associate Professor
Department of Obstetrics and
    Gynecology
Tufts Medical Center
Boston, MA, USA

Hye-Chun Hur, MD, MPH
Minimally Invasive Gynecologic
    Surgeon
Gynecologic Specialty Surgery
Columbia University Irving
    Medical Center
New York, NY, USA

Matthew K. Janssen, MD
Department of Maternal Fetal Medicine
University of Pennsylvania
Philadelphia, PA, USA

Peter Jeppson, MD
Division Chief of Urogynecology
Department of Obstetrics and
    Gynecology
University of New Mexico
Albuquerque, NM, USA

Myrlene Jeudy, MD
Department of Obstetrics and
    Gynecology
Kaiser Permanente
Atlanta, GA, USA

Katherine Johnson, MD
MFM Attending Physician
Department of Obstetrics and
    Gynecology
University of Massachusetts/UMass
    Memorial Medical Center
Worcester, MA, USA

Adina Kern-Goldberger, MD, MPH
Fellow
Department of Obstetrics and
    Gynecology
Hospital of the University of
    Pennsylvania
Philadelphia, PA, USA

Zaraq Khan, MBBS, MCR, FACOG
Chair, Reproductive Endocrinology
    and Infertility
Division of Reproductive
    Endocrinology and Infertility,
    Department of Obstetrics and
    Gynecology
Consultant, Minimally Invasive
    Gynecologic Surgery
Rochester, MN, USA

Tana Kim, MD
Reproductive Endocrinologist
Division of Reproductive
  Endocrinology and Infertility,
  Department of Obstetrics and
  Gynecology
Mayo Clinic
Rochester, MN, USA

Katherine S. Kohari, MD
Assistant Professor
Department of Obstetrics,
  Gynecology, and Reproductive
  Sciences
Section of Maternal-Fetal Medicine
Yale University School of
  Medicine
New Haven, CT, USA

Wendy Kuohung, MD
Associate Professor of Obstetrics and
  Gynecology
Director, Division of Reproductive
  Endocrinology and Infertility
Department of Obstetrics and
  Gynecology
Boston University School
  of Medicine
Boston, MA, USA

Aviva Lee-Parritz, MD
Chief
Department of Obstetrics and
  Gynecology
Boston University
Boston, MA, USA

Peter Lindner, MD
Resident Physician
Department of Obstetrics and
  Gynecology
Walter Reed National Military
  Medical Center
Bethesda, MD, USA

Constance Liu, MD, PhD
Medical Officer
Department of Obstetrics and
  Gynecology
Gallup Indian Medical Center
Gallup, NM, USA

Deirdre J. Lyell, MD
Professor
Department of Obstetrics and
  Gynecology
Stanford University
Palo Alto, CA, USA

Deepali Maheshwari, DO, MPH
Fellow
Department of Obstetrics and
  Gynecology
University of Massachusetts
  Medical School
Worcester, MA, USA

Eliza Rodrigue McElwee, MD
Maternal Fetal Medicine Fellow
Department of Obstetrics and
  Gynecology
Medical University of South Carolina
Charleston, SC, USA

Pooja K. Mehta, MD, MSHP
Women's Health Lead, Cityblock Health
Assistant Professor, Section of
  Community and Population Medicine
Department of Medicine
Louisiana State University Health
  Sciences Center
New Orleans, LA, USA

Magdy Milad, MD, MS
Albert B Gerbie Professor
Department of Obstetrics and
  Gynecology
Northwestern Feinberg School of
  Medicine
Chicago, IL, USA

Jacqueline M. Mills, MD, MPP
Resident Physician
Department of Obstetrics and
    Gynecology
Boston Medical Center
Boston, MA, USA

Rose L. Molina, MD, MPH
Assistant Professor of Obstetrics,
    Gynecology, and Reproductive
    Biology
Department of Obstetrics and
    Gynecology
Beth Israel Deaconess Medical Center
Boston, MA, USA

Samantha Morrison, MD
Chief Resident, PGY4
Department of Obstetrics and
    Gynecology
Crozer-Chester Medical Center
Upland, PA, USA

Laura Newcomb, MD
Department of Obstetrics and
    Gynecology
University of Virginia
Charlottesville, VA, USA

Nyia Noel, MD, MPH
Assistant Professor
Department of Obstetrics and
    Gynecology
Boston University School of Medicine
Boston, MA, USA

Barbara M. O'Brien, MD
Physician
Department of Obstetrics and
    Gynecology
Beth Israel Deaconess Medical Center
Boston, MA, USA

**Alexander Olawaiye, MD, FRCOG,
FACOG, FRCS**
Associate Professor
Department of Obstetrics, Gynecology,
    and Reproductive Sciences
University of Pittsburgh School of
    Medicine
Pittsburgh, PA, USA

Emily A. Oliver, MBBS, MPH
Maternal Fetal Medicine Fellow
Department of Obstetrics and
    Gynecology
Thomas Jefferson University Hospital
Philadelphia, PA, USA

Anna Palatnik, MD
Assistant Professor
Department of Obstetrics and
    Gynecology
Medical College of Wisconsin
Milwaukee, WI, USA

Danielle M. Panelli, MD
Clinical Fellow
Department of Obstetrics and
    Gynecology
Division of Maternal-Fetal Medicine
Stanford University
Stanford, CA, USA

Kristen Pepin, MD, MPH
Assistant Professor
Weill Cornell Medical Center
    New York
New York, NY, USA

Mark Pearlman, MD
Professor, Active Emeritus
Department of Obstetrics and
    Gynecology Department of Surgery
University of Michigan Medical School
Ann Arbor, MI, USA

John Petrozza, MD
Chief, Division of Reproductive
   Medicine & IVF
Department of Obstetrics and
   Gynecology
Massachusetts General Hospital
Boston, MA, USA

Christian M. Pettker, MD
Department of Obstetrics,
   Gynecology, and Reproductive
   Sciences
Yale School of Medicine
New Haven, CT, USA

Nandini Raghuraman, MD, MS
Assistant Professor
Department of Obstetrics and
   Gynecology/Department of
   Surgery
Washington University
St. Louis, MO, USA

Steven J. Ralston, MD, MPH
Chair
Department of Obstetrics and
   Gynecology
Pennsylvania Hospital
Philadelphia, PA, USA

Noah Rindos, MD
Assistant Professor
Department of Obstetrics and
   Gynecology
UPMC Magee-Womens Hospital
Pittsburgh, PA, USA

Nick Rockefeller, MD
Clinical Fellow
Female Pelvic Medicine and
   Reconstructive Surgery
University of New Mexico
Albuquerque, NM, USA

Amanda Roman-Camargo, MD
Associate Professor
Department of Obstetrics and
   Gynecology
Thomas Jefferson University
Philadelphia, PA, USA

Stephanie Rothenberg, MD
Pacific NW Fertility
Seattle, WA, USA

Caitlin Sacha, MD
Clinical Research Fellow in
   Reproductive Endocrinology and
   Infertility
Department of Obstetrics and
   Gynecology, Massachusetts
   General Hospital
Harvard Medical School
Boston, MA, USA

Maryl Sackeim, MD
Faculty
Family Planning Division
Kaiser Permanente San Francisco
San Francisco, CA, USA

Joseph Sanfilippo, MD
Department of Obstetrics and
   Gynecology
UPMC Magee-Womens Hospital
Pittsburgh, PA, USA

Lauren D. Schiff, MD
Assistant Professor of Minimally
   Invasive Gynecologic Surgery
Department of Obstetrics and
   Gynecology
University of North Carolina School
   of Medicine
Chapel Hill, NC, USA

Elizabeth B. Schmidt, MD, MSCI, FACOG, FACS
Chief of Family Planning
Department of Obstetrics and
  Gynecology
Northwell
Great Neck, NY, USA

Sierra J. Seaman, MD
Physician
Department of Obstetrics and
  Gynecology
Columbia University Irving Medical
  Center—New York Presbyterian
  Hospital
New York, NY, USA

Neel Shah, MD, MPP
Assistant Professor
Department of Obstetrics,
  Gynecology, and Reproductive
  Biology
Harvard Medical School
Boston, MA, USA

Scott A. Shainker, DO, MS
The Annie and Chase Koch Chair in
  Obstetrics and Gynecology
Assistant Professor of Obstetrics,
  Gynecology, and Reproductive
  Biology
Beth Israel Deaconess Medical Center/
  Harvard Medical School
Boston, MA, USA

Alireza A. Shamshirsaz, MD
Associate Professor, Fetal surgeon/
  Maternal Fetal Medicine
Chair, Fetal Center Steering Committee
Chief, Division of Fetal Therapy and
  Surgery

Director, Fetal Surgery Fellowship
Co-Chief, Maternal Fetal Surgery
  Section
Department of Obstetrics and
  Gynecology/Department of
  Surgery
Baylor College of Medicine
Children's Fetal Center, Texas
  Children's Hospital
Houston, TX, USA

Laura Smith, MD
Clinical Fellow
Department of Obstetrics and
  Gynecology
Beth Israel Deaconess Medical Center
Boston, MA, USA

Ellen Solomon, MD
Assistant Professor of Obstetrics and
  Gynecology
Division of Urogynecology and Pelvic
  Surgery
University of Massachusetts, Baystate
  Medical Center
Springfield, MA, USA

Melissa H. Spiel, DO
Assistant Professor
Department of Obstetrics, Gynecology,
  and Reproductive Biology
Harvard Medical School
Boston, MA, USA

Elizabeth A. Stier, MD
Professor
Department of Obstetrics and
  Gynecology
Boston University School of
  Medicine
Boston, MA, USA

Julie Stone, MD
Fellow
Department of Maternal Fetal Medicine
Tufts Medical Center
Boston, MA, USA

Leanna Sudhof, MD
Attending Physician
Department of Obstetrics and
    Gynecology
Beth Israel Deaconess Medical Center
Boston, MA, USA

Monique Swain, MD
Assistant Professor
Department of Obstetrics and
    Gynecology
Henry Ford Hospital
Detroit, MI, USA

Sarah E. Taylor, MD
Assistant Professor of Gynecologic
    Oncology
Department of Obstetrics, Gynecology,
    and Reproductive Sciences
Pittsburgh, PA, USA

Jessica Traylor, MD
Physician
Department of Obstetrics and
    Gynecology
Northwestern University Feinberg
    School of Medicine
Chicago, IL, USA

Susan Tsai, MD
Assistant Professor
Department of Obstetrics and
    Gynecology
Northwestern University Feinberg
    School of Medicine
Chicago, IL, USA

Paul Tyan, MD, MSCR
Obstetrics and Gynecology Physician
Department of Obstetrics and
    Gynecology
Capital Women's Care
Leesburg, VA

Judith Volkar, MD
Assistant Professor
University of Pittsburgh
    Medical School
Pittsburgh, PA, USA

Neeta L. Vora, MD
Associate Professor
Department of Obstetrics and
    Gynecology
University of North Carolina
Chapel Hill, NC, USA

Megan Wasson, DO
Associate Professor of Obstetrics and
    Gynecology
Chair of the Department of Medical
    and Surgical Gynecology
Mayo Clinic in Arizona
Phoenix, AZ, USA

Blair J. Wylie, MD, MPH
Director, Division of Maternal Fetal
    Medicine
Department of Obstetrics and
    Gynecology
Beth Israel Deaconess Medical
    Center
Boston, MA, USA

Johnny Yi, MD
Department of Medical and Surgical
    Gynecology
Mayo Clinic Arizona
Phoenix, AZ, USA

Brett C. Young, MD
Attending
Department of Obstetrics and
    Gynecology
Beth Israel Deaconess Medical
    Center
Boston, MA, USA

Mandy Yunker, DO, MSCR
Associate Professor
Department of Obstetrics and
    Gynecology
Vanderbilt Medical Center
Nashville, TN, USA

Chloe Zera, MD, MPH
Assistant Professor
Department of Maternal Fetal Medicine,
    Obstetrics and Gynecology
Beth Israel Deaconess Medical
    Center/Harvard Medical School
Boston, MA, USA

John Zupancic, MD, ScD
Associate Chief of Neonatology
Department of Neonatology
Beth Israel Deaconess Medical
    Center
Boston, MA, USA

Magnesium Sulphate for Seizure Prophylaxis in Women With Preeclampsia

The MAGPIE Trial

PETER LINDNER AND SHAD DEERING

"Magnesium sulphate halves the risk of eclampsia, and probably reduces the risk of maternal death. There do not appear to be substantive harmful effects to mother or baby in the short term."

—THE MAGPIE TRIAL COLLABORATIVE GROUP[1]

Research Question: Do women with preeclampsia and their babies benefit from magnesium sulphate?[1]

Funding: UK Medical Research Council, UK Department for International Development, UNDP/UNFPA/WHO/World Bank Special Programme of Research, Development and Research Training in Human Reproduction

Year Study Began: 1998

Year Study Published: 2002

Study Location: 33 countries

Who Was Studied: Pregnant women with singleton or multiple gestations with preeclampsia (blood pressure >140mmHg systolic and/or >90 mmHg diastolic on 2 separate occasions with documented proteinuria) who had not yet delivered or were less than 24-hours postpartum.

Who Was Excluded: Patients with a known hypersensitivity to magnesium, history of myasthenia gravis or those in a hepatic coma at risk of renal failure were excluded.

How Many Patients: 10,141

Study Overview: This was a randomized, double-blind, placebo-controlled trial. See Figure 1.1

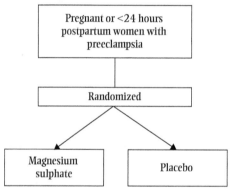

Figure 1.1. Study overview: MAGPIE Trial

Study Intervention: Patients were randomized to receive a loading dose of either magnesium sulphate or placebo, followed by 24 hours of maintenance therapy of the same.

Magnesium toxicity was evaluated by serial reflex exams every 30 minutes and urine output monitored hourly. Magnesium dosing was reduced by half when there was evidence of toxicity or low urine output. If a patient had an eclamptic seizure the trial treatment was stopped and nontrial magnesium sulphate was started.

Follow-Up: Until discharge from the hospital

Endpoints: Primary outcomes: eclampsia, fetal death. Secondary outcomes: Significant maternal morbidity (as individual, prespecified outcomes and as a composite), complications of labor including cesarean section, and neonatal morbidity.

RESULTS

- In the magnesium sulphate group, there was a 58% risk reduction of eclampsia when compared to the placebo arm. The number needed to treat to prevent an eclamptic seizure in women with severe preeclampsia was 63, and 109 for mild preeclampsia.
- There was no difference in the risk of maternal death between the two groups (relative risk [RR]: 0.55, 95% confidence interval [CI]: 0.26–1.14). Magnesium sulphate did not affect maternal morbidity compared to the placebo when evaluating for respiratory depression, respiratory arrest, pulmonary edema, cardiac arrest, renal failure, or liver failure.
- There was a lower risk of placental abruption in patients who received magnesium sulphate prior to delivery. The article cites 12 fewer placental abruptions per 1000 women.
- Women who received magnesium sulphate during the labor process were noted to have a 5% higher risk of requiring a cesarean section (RR 1.05, 95% CI 1.00–1.11, $p = 0.02$).
- There was no difference in length of hospital stay or need for admission to an intensive care unit between the placebo and magnesium groups.
- There was no difference in the in utero or neonatal death rate between the 2 groups (RR: 1.02, 95% CI: 0.92–1.14).
- There was no difference in effectiveness of magnesium sulphate when comparing intramuscular versus intravenous routes of administration. (See Table 1.1.)

Table 1.1. SUMMARY OF MAGPIE TRIAL'S KEY FINDINGS

Outcome	Magnesium Sulphate Arm (%)	Placebo Arm (%)	p-value	Relative Risk (95% confidence interval)
Eclamptic convulsion	0.8	1.9	<0.0001	0.42 (0.29–0.60)
Eclamptic convulsions in severe preeclampsia	1.2	2.8	Not given	0.42 (0.23–0.76)
Eclamptic convulsions in mild preeclampsia	0.7	1.6	Not given	0.42 (0.26–0.67)
Any serious maternal morbidity	3.9	3.6	Not given	Not given
Maternal mortality	0.2	0.4	0.11	Not given
Fetal death	12.7	12.4	Not given	1.02 (0.92–1.14)
Cesarean delivery	50	48.0	0.02	Not given

Criticisms and Limitations: The most important limitation of this study is the evolving definition of preeclampsia with and without severe features. The Magpie study utilizes a classic definition of preeclampsia. Blood pressure parameters and definitions of proteinuria have changed slightly since then, as have qualifying laboratory and clinical characteristics that classify a patient as severe. Despite these newer definitions, the benefits of magnesium remain steadfast, and the therapy is still considered first-line treatment in the prevention of eclampsia in women with preeclampsia.

Although the Magpie trial is a large, multicenter, randomized controlled trial, the magnesium sulphate arm had a significantly higher rate of maternal side effects such as hot flashes and nausea. Therefore, the presence of these side effects could have inadvertently unblinded the study. It is estimated that approximately 20% of the women allocated magnesium sulphate were able to determine which treatment they were receiving. The clinical significance of this remains unknown.

The study did not randomize route of administration for magnesium; therefore, the assumptions made about equipoise between intramuscular and intravenous routes of magnesium should be considered with caution; however, both routes were used, and it is reasonable to consider the intramuscular route in the developing world or in clinical scenarios where intravenous access is not available.

Other Relevant Studies and Information:

- A follow-up study by the Magpie Collaborative Group evaluated long-term maternal and neonatal effects 2 years after receiving magnesium sulphate. There was no increase in the risk of death or disability.[2]
- A meta-analysis that evaluated randomized control trials that compared magnesium sulphate with either a placebo or other anticonvulsants was published in 2010. The study came to similar conclusions as the Magpie trial.[3]
- Current American College of Obstetricians and Gynecologists (ACOG) guidelines recommend magnesium sulphate for preeclampsia with severe features as well as in patients with severe gestational hypertension.[4,5]
- The Magpie study demonstrated that magnesium sulfate reduces eclamptic seizure in patients with mild preeclampsia. However, subsequent review of available trials do not demonstrate a clear improvement in maternal or fetal outcomes in this cohort[6]; thus, ACOG guidelines do not currently support the universal use of magnesium sulfate in preeclampsia without severe features.[5]

Summary and Implications: Magnesium sulphate therapy reduces the risk of eclampsia by 58% without increasing maternal or fetal morbidity.

CLINICAL CASE: POSTPARTUM MAGNESIUM SULPHATE THERAPY FOR SEIZURE PROPHYLAXIS

Case History

A 37-year-old G2P1001 at 39+0 weeks estimated gestational age was admitted to labor and delivery in active labor. Upon assessment she is complaining of a severe headache that has not resolved despite pain medications and vital signs demonstrate persistent systolic blood pressure greater than 170 mmHg. Her prenatal course was complicated by gestational hypertension, and this pregnancy was conceived with the aid of in vitro fertilization.

Based on the findings of the Magpie trial, how should this patient be treated?

Suggested Answer

Initiation of magnesium sulfate is considered standard of care for patients with hypertensive diseases of pregnancy with severe features. In this case, the patient has severe range hypertension and a persistent headache. The Magpie trial demonstrated a reduced risk of eclamptic convulsions with magnesium sulfate. There is no difference in the efficacy of intramuscular magnesium sulphate versus intravenous administration, but intravenous administration is preferred due to irritation with intramuscular administration. In addition to initiating magnesium sulphate, prompt anti-hypertensive therapy should be initiated in this scenario.

References

1. Altman D, Carroli G, Duley L, Farrell B, Moodley J, Neilson J, Smith D; Magpie Trial Collaboration Group. Do women with pre-eclampsia, and their babies, benefit from magnesium sulphate? The Magpie Trial: a randomised placebo-controlled trial. *Lancet* 2002 Jun 1;359(9321):1877–1890. doi:10.1016/s0140-6736(02)08778-0. PMID:12057549.
2. Magpie Trial Follow-Up Study Collaborative Group. The Magpie trial: a randomized trial comparing magnesium sulphate with placebo for pre-eclampsia. Outcome for women at 2 years. *BJOG* 2007;114:300–309.
3. Duley L, Gülmezoglu AM, Henderson-Smart DJ, Chou D. Magnesium sulphate and other anticonvulsants for women with pre-eclampsia. *Cochrane Database Sys Rev.* 2010;11:CD000025.

4. American College of Obstetricians and Gynecologists, College of Obstetricians and Gynecologists, Task Force on Hypertension in Pregnancy, Force on Hypertension in Pregnancy, Task Force on Hypertension in Pregnancy, American College of Obstetricians and Gynecologists. Hypertension in pregnancy. Report of the American College of Obstetricians and Gynecologists' Task Force on Hypertension in Pregnancy. *Obstetrics Gynecol.* 2013;122:1122–1131.

5. Gestational Hypertension and Preeclampsia. ACOG Practice Bulletin No. 202. American College of Obstetricians and Gynecologists. *Obstet Gynecol.* 2019; 133:el–e25.

6. Sibai BM. Magnesium sulfate prophylaxis in preeclampsia: lessons learned from recent trials. *Am J Obstet Gynecol.* 2004;190(6):1520–1526. Review. PubMed PMID: 15284724.

2

Low-Dose Aspirin for the Prevention and Treatment of Preeclampsia

The CLASP Trial

DANIELLE M. PANELLI AND DEIRDRE J. LYELL

"Low-dose aspirin may be justified in women judged to be especially liable to early-onset pre-eclampsia severe enough to need very preterm delivery."

—CLASP (COLLABORATIVE LOW-DOSE ASPIRIN
STUDY IN PREGNANCY) COLLABORATIVE GROUP[1]

Research Question: Does maternal antiplatelet therapy during pregnancy decrease the risk of preeclampsia? Secondarily, what are the impacts of aspirin use on duration of pregnancy, maternal hemorrhage, intrauterine growth restriction, and other maternal and neonatal outcomes?

Year Published: 1994

Funding: The study was commercially sponsored by the Clinical Trial Service Unit and the Radcliffe Infirmary switchboard, the UK Medical Research Council, Sterling Winthrop, Bayer-Europe, and the European Aspirin Foundation. The authors report that the project was completed independently of the commercial sponsors with the exception of medication donation.

Years of Study: Women were recruited between January 1988 and December 1992.

Study Location: 213 centers in 16 countries.

Who Was Studied: Women between 12 and 32 weeks of gestation deemed to be at risk of either preeclampsia or intrauterine growth restriction (IUGR) during the index pregnancy. Patients either had a history of preeclampsia or IUGR in a prior pregnancy, chronic hypertension, renal disease, advanced maternal age, "family history," or multiple pregnancy and were thus candidates for prophylactic treatment or had preeclampsia or IUGR in the current pregnancy and were considered candidates for therapeutic treatment.

Who Was Excluded: Women with an increased risk of bleeding or asthma, an allergy to aspirin, or a high likelihood of imminent delivery.

How Many Patients: 9,364

Study Overview: This was a randomized, double-blind, placebo-controlled trial. See Figure 2.1

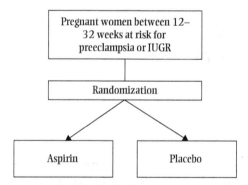

Figure 2.1. Study overview: the CLASP Trial

After the study was initiated, recruitment goals were expanded to 10,000 (originally 4,000) in order to better be able to detect a 25% decrease in the rare event of stillbirth or neonatal death. The study had originally only been powered to detect a 25% decrease in the development of preeclampsia, a 100g increase in birth weight, and an increase of 1 day in mean duration of gestation.

Study Intervention: Women were randomized to treatment with 60 mg aspirin daily versus a matching placebo tablet. This dose was chosen as it was thought to balance side effects and effective inhibition of maternal cyclo-oxygenase-dependent platelet aggregation.

Follow-Up: 6 weeks postpartum

Endpoints: Primary outcome: a composite of development of proteinuric pree-clampsia, IUGR, 100g birthweight difference, and 1 day difference in gestational age at delivery. Secondary outcome: maternal or neonatal bleeding event, still-birth or neonatal demise.

RESULTS

- A total of 6.7% of women randomized to aspirin developed proteinuric preeclampsia versus 7.6% of those assigned to the placebo group. This corresponds to a nonsignificant 12% decrease in the odds of developing preeclampsia among women who received aspirin. There was a 22% reduction among those in the "prophylaxis" arm who entered the study prior to 20 weeks gestation ($p = 0.06$).
- Women who received aspirin were significantly less likely to deliver before 37 weeks than women who received placebo (19.7% vs. 22%, $p = 0.003$).
- The mean neonatal birthweight from the aspirin group was 32g greater than that of the control group ($p = 0.05$), but there was no significant difference in IUGR rates.
- There were no significant differences in stillbirths, neonatal deaths, abruption, antepartum hemorrhage, neonatal intraventricular hemorrhage, or adverse maternal experiences with neuraxial anesthesia. (See Table 2.1.)

Table 2.1. STUDY OUTCOMES

	Outcome	Placebo (%)	Aspirin (%)	Odds Reduction
Prophylactic Group	Proteinuric preeclampsia	7.6	6.7	13% reduction (NS)
	Preterm delivery	19.1	17.2	12% reduction ($p = 0.03$)
Therapeutic Group	Proteiniuric preeclampsia	7.5	6.9	8% reduction (NS)
	Preterm delivery	22.2	19.7	21% reduction ($p = 0.03$)

Abbreviation: NS, nonsignificant.

Criticisms and Limitations: Postpartum follow-up information was only available on 8,915 women; of these, only 66% achieved at least 95% medication adherence. In addition, this trial was powered to detect only a 25% decrease in stillbirth and neonatal death and as a result had limited ability to detect smaller degrees of change in these rare outcomes. In addition, this study included two distinct subpopulations: those receiving prophylactic aspirin and those receiving therapeutic aspirin. Aspirin may have a differential impact on these two groups; however, this study was not adequately powered to examine the impact on each subpopulation alone.

Other Relevant Studies and Information:

- In recent years, higher doses of aspirin, up to 150 mg, have been shown to be associated with greater reductions in preeclampsia rates.[2,3]
- Several meta-analyses have been published evaluating the dose and timing of initiation of aspirin to elucidate optimal benefit. While results have been conflicting, there is some evidence to support additional value in initiation of aspirin prior to 16 weeks gestation.[2–5]
- The safety of prophylactic aspirin has been affirmed; a US Preventive Services Task Force (USPTF) review found no increase in placental abruption, postpartum hemorrhage, or mean blood loss.[6] Several reviews have also affirmed fetal safety, with no demonstrated increase in fetal anomalies, ductal closure, or intracranial hemorrhage. The American College of Obstetricians and Gynecologists (ACOG) states that the data suggesting gastroschisis to be twice as common in women with aspirin exposure should be interpreted with extreme caution.[7]
- The authors cautioned that the results of the CLASP trial justified the use of prophylactic aspirin only in women who are at particular risk of early-onset pre-eclampsia (before 32 weeks), but available evidence and safety data since CLASP supports broader application of prophylactic aspirin to women with moderate risk factors.
- Current recommendations include 81mg aspirin for women at high risk for the development of preeclampsia and those with multiple moderate risk factors that likely have compounding risk effect.[8]

Summary and Implications: This study failed to demonstrate significant differences in the development of preeclampsia, stillbirth, or neonatal demise with 60mg aspirin use versus placebo but did identify a trend toward a lower incidence of preeclampsia at earlier gestational ages. Based on the results from the CLASP trial and several other studies, the USPTF and ACOG guidelines currently recommend initiating aspirin therapy after 12 weeks gestation to all women considered to be at high risk for developing preeclampsia.[6-7]

CLINICAL CASE

Case History

A 29-year-old healthy G3P1 presents for her first prenatal visit at 12 weeks gestation. She has a history of preeclampsia with severe features in a pregnancy two years ago, which required delivery at 34 weeks. She is worried about recurrence of this disease. How would you counsel her regarding antepartum management?

Suggested Answer

Based on USPTF and ACOG guidelines, this patient should be offered daily aspirin after 12 weeks of gestation (ideally before 16 weeks), as this has been shown to reduce rates of preeclampsia and need for preterm delivery as per the results of CLASP trial and other studies that drive this recommendation. At this time, both guidelines recommend a dose of 81mg.

References

1. CLASP: a randomised trial of low-dose aspirin for the prevention and treatment of pre-eclampsia among 9364 pregnant women. CLASP (Collaborative Low-dose Aspirin Study in Pregnancy) Collaborative Group. *Lancet.* 1994 Mar 12;343(8898):619–629. PMID:7906809.
2. Rolnik DL et al. Aspirin versus placebo in pregnancies at high risk for preterm preeclampsia. *NEJM.* 2017;377(7): 613–622.
3. McMaster-Fay RA, Hyett JA. Comment on: preventing preeclampsia with aspirin: does dose or timing matter? *Am J Obstet Gynecol.* 2017;217(3):383.
4. Roberge S, Nicolaides K, Demers S, Hyett J, Chaillet N, Bujold E. The role of aspirin dose on the prevention of preeclampsia and fetal growth restriction: systematic review and meta-analysis. *Am J Obstet Gynecol.* 2017;216(2):110–120.
5. Meher S, Duley L, Hunter K, Askie L. Antiplatelet therapy before or after 16 weeks' gestation for preventing preeclampsia: an individual participant data meta-analysis. *Am J Obstet Gynecol.* 2017;216(2):121–128.
6. Final update summary: low-dose aspirin use for the prevention of morbidity and mortality from preeclampsia: preventive medication. U.S. Preventive Services Task Force. September 2016.
7. Gyamfi-Bannerman C, Manuck T. Low-dose aspirin use during pregnancy. *ACOG Comm Opin 743.* 2018;132(1):44–52.

8. Henderson JT, Whitlock EP, O'Connor E, Senger CA, Thompson JH, Rowland MG. Low-dose aspirin for the prevention of morbidity and mortality from preeclampsia: a systematic evidence review for the U.S. Preventive Services Task Force. Evidence Synthesis No. 112. AHRQ Publication No. 14–05207-EF-1. Rockville, MD: Agency for Healthcare Research and Quality; 2014.

3

First Trimester Hemoglobin A1 and Risk for Major Malformation and Spontaneous Abortion

RACHEL BLAKE AND CHLOE ZERA

"Although the risks for both adverse outcomes were markedly elevated following a first trimester in very poor metabolic control, there was a broad range of control over which the risks were not substantially elevated."

—GREENE ET AL.[1]

Research Question: Among women with diabetes, is glycemic control in early pregnancy associated with congenital malformation?

Funding: Not reported

Year Study Began: 1983

Year Study Published: 1989

Study Location: Joslin Diabetes Center and Brigham and Women's Hospital Boston, MA

Who Was Studied: All patients with insulin-dependent diabetes presenting at or before 12 weeks of gestation

Who Was Excluded: Patients with incomplete outcomes data ($N = 21$)

How Many Patients: 303

Study Overview: This was a prospective study examining the relationship between first trimester glycosylated hemoglobin A1 levels in patients with pre-existing insulin-controlled diabetes. See Figure 3.1

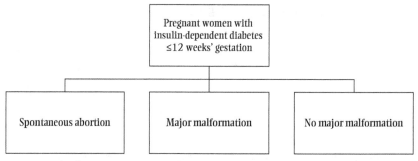

Figure 3.1. Study overview

Routine ultrasounds were performed on all patients by one author who was blinded to first trimester HbA1 value. First trimester spontaneous abortion was defined as serial ultrasound demonstrating empty intrauterine gestational sac or fetus without cardiac motion or histologic identification of trophoblast. Malformations were considered major if they were fatal, required surgery, or had significant "anatomic or cosmetic" impact.

Parametric tests were used to calculate the risk ratios for spontaneous abortion and major malformations stratified by first trimester HbA1.

Follow-Up: Congenital anomalies assessed by clinical examination prior to newborn hospital discharge; for subjects with heart murmur identified on newborn exam, there was a follow-up call to the patient or pediatrician to determine whether a cardiac anomaly was identified post-discharge.

Endpoints: Primary outcomes were first-trimester spontaneous abortion, and major congenital malformation (fatal, required surgery to correct, or were of major anatomic or cosmetic importance).

RESULTS

- Thirty-five percent of the total patient population had a first trimester HbA1 greater than 9 standard deviations above the mean, and 14% were above 12 standard deviations above the mean. (See Table 3.1.)
- Ten patients were lost to follow-up (mean HbA1 12.0%), and nine patients were known to have transferred their care to other physicians during the study period (mean HbA1 9.6%).
- There were a total of 20 major malformations diagnosed, of which 8 were considered "fatal." Five of those patients elected termination.
- The most common major fatal malformations were Tetralogy of Fallot, anencephaly, and diaphragmatic hernia. The most common nonfatal malformations were ventricular septal defect, unilateral renal agenesis, and anomalous vertebrae.
- There were no differences in maternal age, White classification, or diabetes score between those with a fetal malformation or spontaneous abortion and those without.
- The mean HbA1 value was significantly lower ($p < 0.005$) among patients in the no major malformations group (9.9%) compared to that of the major malformations (12.4%) and spontaneous abortion group (11.6%). There was no significant difference between the HbA1 levels of patients with major malformations (12.4%) compared to patients with spontaneous abortions (11.6%).
- There was an association of HbA1 with risk for spontaneous abortion, particularly ≥11.1%.
- The risk for major malformations was also associated with HbA1 ≥12.8%.

Table 3.1. RESULTS

First Trimester HbA1 (%)	Approximate HbA1c (%) (James 1981)	Risk Ratio (95% CI) for Spontaneous Abortion	Risk Ratio (95% CI) for Major Malformation
<9.3	6.5	1.0 (ref)	1.0 (ref)
9.4–11.0	6.6–7.9	0.7 (0.3–1.6)	1.7 (0.4–1.7)
11.1–12.7	8.0–9.3	1.98 (1.03–3.38)	1.4 (0.3–8.3)
12.8–14.4	9.4–-10.8	2.9 (1.4–5.8)	12.8 (4.7–35.0)
>14.4	>10.8	3.0 (1.3–7.0)	13.2 (4.3–40.4)

Criticisms and Limitations: There is likely a bias toward patients with relatively well-controlled diabetes in this cohort, suggested by the mean HbA1 of 12% among patients lost to follow-up. Outcome ascertainment may also have been biased, as women who experienced miscarriage prior to establishing care were not enrolled, and determination of malformations was limited to prenatal ultrasound and neonatal exam, with limited infant follow-up.

This study does not include a control group without diabetes, therefore one cannot compare the risk of malformation or spontaneous abortion between patients with well-controlled diabetes and those without diabetes. Finally, there was no adjustment for confounders that are known to be associated with risk for pregnancy loss and/or congenital anomalies, including maternal obesity, smoking, and age.

Interpretation of the findings must also be placed in the context of the era during which this study was conducted. Advances in ultrasound have allowed for much earlier identification of first trimester pregnancy as well as early assessment of fetal anatomy. The standard of care for ultrasound-identified structural abnormalities now includes prenatal diagnosis with microarray, whereas in this study, only one amniocentesis is mentioned. Notably, this amniocentesis (performed for advanced maternal age) identified a fetus with Turner's syndrome, which was included in the group with first trimester losses for the purposes of analysis. It is possible that more genetic and/or structural abnormalities would have been identified in current clinical practice.

Other Relevant Studies and Information:

- While early work was conflicting, the majority of data have demonstrated a correlation between diabetes control in the first trimester and risk for both spontaneous abortions and major malformations. A small study showed that the mean glycated hemoglobin A1 concentrations of women with diabetes were higher among those with spontaneous abortions than that of women who had continuing pregnancies.[2]
- Several studies have found that initial glycohemoglobin concentrations in pregnancy above 12% or median first-trimester preprandial glucose concentrations above 120 mg/dL are associated with increased risk when compared to that of women without diabetes.[3,4]
- The American Diabetes Associations recommends a prepregnancy A1C of <6.5% to reduce the risk of congenital anomalies and other complications.[5] The American College of Obstetricians and Gynecologists recommends maintaining glucose control near "physiologic levels" before and throughout pregnancy for the same reason.[6]

- Interestingly, numerous studies have demonstrated that the degree of metabolic control necessary to prevent spontaneous abortions is greater than that required to avoid major malformations; however, the risk of either event likely increases in proportion to the degree of blood sugar elevation.[7, 8] Glycemic control in the weeks surrounding conception seems to be most important with respect to risk for spontaneous abortion.[9] Nonetheless, in all of these studies, normal outcomes were seen in women with a wide range of glycemic control.[10]
- Of note, this study uses Hemoglobin A1, which is the first fraction to separate on cation exchange chromatography. Subsequent fractions are designated HbA_{1a}, HbA_{1b}, and HbA_{1c}, respective of their order of elution. Hemoglobin a1c is currently more commonly used as a measure of blood sugar control; HgA1 and hga1c are correlated, but HgA1 generally demonstrates a higher value than the equivalent hemoglobin a1c.[11]

Summary and Implications: Despite some limitations, this study demonstrated an association of major malformations and spontaneous abortions with degree of glycemic control in the first trimester of pregnancy. Current guidelines from the American Diabetes Association recommend that women target a normal hemoglobin A1c (<6.5) prior to pregnancy.[9]

CLINICAL CASE: FIRST TRIMESTER HBA1 AND RISK FOR FETAL MALFORMATIONS AND SPONTANEOUS ABORTION

Case History

A 34-year-old G1 with type 1 diabetes presents to your office at 8 weeks gestation with an unplanned but desired pregnancy. She is concerned about her risk for miscarriage and fetal congenital anomalies, because her HbA1c drawn last week at her endocrinologist's office was 8.5%. You look at her continuous glucose monitor download with her and note that her blood sugars have been within her target range since she adjusted her pump settings at that visit. She asks you if could estimate her risk of having a major congenital defect since she is aware that her risk might be higher than average.

Suggested Answer

This study, like many others, does show an association with risk for pregnancy loss and congenital anomalies with elevated first trimester HbA1 values. However, it is important to note that most women had normal pregnancies, even within a cohort of women with a wide range of HbA1. These data do not allow us to estimate what percentage of adverse pregnancy outcomes should be considered a result of glycemic control alone, as there are miscarriages and congenital anomalies among women with diabetes that are not attributable to glycemic control and therefore may even overestimate her individual risk.

It is important when counseling women with diabetes that while they are at risk for adverse pregnancy outcomes, the majority of women have normal pregnancies. Even in unplanned pregnancies in which glycemic control is suboptimal prior to conception, good glycemic control in the late first trimester may modify the risk for structural anomalies. A multidisciplinary approach to optimizing the care for women with diabetes often results in healthy pregnancies with term delivery.

References

1. Greene MF, Hare JW, Cloherty JP, Benacerraf BR, Soeldner JS. First-trimester hemoglobin A1 and risk for major malformation and spontaneous abortion in diabetic pregnancy. *Teratology*. 1989 Mar;39(3):225–231. doi:10.1002/tera.1420390303. PMID:2727930.
2. Miodovnik M, Mimouni F, Tsang RC, Ammar E, Kaplan L, Siddiqi TA. Glycemic control and spontaneous abortion in insulin-dependent diabetic women. *Obstet Gynecol*. 1986 Sep;68(3):366–369.
3. Miodovnik M, Skillman C, Holroyde JC, Butler JB, Wendel JS, Siddiqi TA. Elevated maternal glycohemoglobin in early pregnancy and spontaneous abortion among insulin-dependent diabetic women. *Am J Obstet Gynecol*. 1985 Oct 15;153(4):439–442.
4. Rosenn B, Miodovnik M, Combs CA, Khoury J, Siddiqi TA. Glycemic thresholds for spontaneous abortion and congenital malformations in insulin-dependent diabetes mellitus. *Obstet Gynecol*. 1994 Oct;84(4):515–520.
5. American Diabetes Association. 14. Management of Diabetes in Pregnancy: Standards of Medical Care in Diabetes-2020. *Diabetes Care*. 2020 Jan;43(Suppl 1):S183–S192. doi:10.2337/dc20-S014. PMID:31862757.
6. American College of Obstetricians and Gynecologists' Committee on Practice Bulletins—Obstetrics. ACOG Practice Bulletin No. 201: Pregestational Diabetes Mellitus. *Obstet Gynecol*. 2018;132(6):e228–e248. doi:10.1097/AOG.0000000000002960
7. Greene MF. Spontaneous abortions and major malformations in women with diabetes mellitus. *Semin Reprod Endocrinol*. 1999;17(2):127–136.

8. Combs CA, Kitzmiller JL. Spontaneous abortion and congenital malformations in diabetes. *Baillieres Clin Obstet Gynaecol.* 1991 Jun;5(2):315–331.

9. Miodovnik, M. Preconceptional metabolic status and risk for spontaneous abortion in insulin-dependent diabetic pregnancies. *Am J Perinatol.* 1988 Oct;5(4):368–373.

10. Langer O. A spectrum of glucose thresholds may effectively prevent complications in the pregnant diabetic patient. *Semin Perinatol.* 2002 Jun;26(3):196–205.

11. Peterson KP, Pavlovich JG, Goldstein D, Little R, England J, Peterson CM. What is hemoglobin A1c? An analysis of glycated hemoglobins by electrospray ionization mass spectrometry. *Clin Chemistry.* 1998;44(9):1951–1958. PMID 9732983

4

Effect of Treatment of Gestational Diabetes Mellitus on Pregnancy Outcomes

The ACHOIS Trial

ALEXANDRA BELCHER-OBEJERO-PAZ AND
AVIVA LEE-PARRITZ

"Our results indicate that treatment of gestational diabetes in the form of dietary advice, blood glucose monitoring, and insulin therapy as required for glycemic control reduces the rate of serious perinatal complications without increasing the risk of cesarean delivery."

—ACHOIS TRIAL GROUP[1]

Research Question: Does the treatment of woman with gestational diabetes reduce the risk of perinatal complications and affect maternal outcomes, mood, and quality of life?

Funding: National Health and Medical Research Council Australia, the Queen Victoria Hospital Research Foundation

Year Study Began: 1993

Year Study Published: 2005

Study Location: 18 sites in Australia and the United Kingdom

Who Was Studied: Patients with singleton or twin pregnancy between 16 and 30 weeks gestation with a glycemic response to a standard oral glucose-tolerance test that was intermediate between the normal and diabetic response, defined as (1) having one or more factors for gestational diabetes *or* (2) a positive 50-g oral glucose challenge test (>140mg/dL after 1 hour) and having a 75-g oral glucose tolerance test with a 2-hour value of >140mg/dL to <190mg/dL.

Who Was Excluded: Patients with previously treated gestational diabetes, a glycemic response indicating diabetes, or active chronic systemic disease (with the exception of essential hypertensive disease).

How Many Patients: 1,000

Study Overview: See Figure 4.1

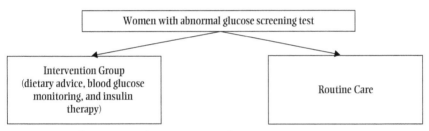

Figure 4.1 Study overview: the ACHOIS Trial

Study Intervention: Patients were randomized to either the intervention group or routine care. Interventions included dietary advice from a qualified dietitian and instruction on how to self-monitor glucose levels 4 times daily until they reached target ranges for 2 weeks. Insulin therapy was initiated based on elevated glucose levels. Patients in the routine care group and their caregivers were not informed of the diagnosis of glucose intolerance of pregnancy and were not provided with intervention or treatment, replicating the standard of care at the time.

Follow-Up: Enrollment (approximately 29 weeks gestational age) until 3 months postpartum

Endpoints: Primary infant outcomes: Serious perinatal injury (i.e., death, shoulder dystocia, bone fracture, and nerve palsy), admission to the neonatal nursery, and jaundice requiring phototherapy. Primary maternal outcomes: the need for induction of labor, the need for cesarean birth, maternal physical and mental health status. Secondary infant outcomes: gestational age at birth, birth weight and other measures of health. Maternal secondary outcomes: mode of delivery, maternal weight gain, number antenatal admissions, and other complications.

RESULTS

- Rates of serious perinatal outcomes were significantly lower in the intervention group (1%) compared to the routine care group (4%). However, rates of admission to the neonatal nursery were significantly higher among women in the intervention group (71%) than the routine care group (61%). Infants in the intervention group were less likely to be large for gestational age, and less likely to be macrosomic (both p <0.001). (See Table 4.1.)
- Infants born to mothers in the intervention group had lower birth weights when compared to those who receive routine care (p <0.0001) and were born at earlier gestational ages (p =0.01). In addition, they were more likely to undergo induction of labor (p <0.001).
- Treatment of gestational diabetes did not have any effect on the need for treating neonatal hypoglycemia.

Table 4.1. SUMMARY OF INFANT AND MATERNAL PRIMARY AND SECONDARY CLINICAL OUTCOMES IN ACHOIS STUDY

Outcome	Intervention Group (n = 506)	Routine Care Group (n = 524)	Adjusted p-value[a]
Neonatal			
Any serious perinatal outcome[b]	7 (1%)	23 (4%)	0.01
Death	0 (0%)	5 (1%)	0.07
Birth weight in g (±SD)	3335±551	3482±660	<0.001
Macrosomia[c]	49 (10%)	110 (21%)	<0.001
Maternal			
Induction of labor	189 (39%)	150 (29%)	<0.001
Cesarean delivery	152 (31%)	164 (32%)	0.73
Weight gain in kg (±SD)	8.1±0.3	9.8±0.4	0.01
Preeclampsia	58 (12%)	93 (18%)	0.02

[a]Adjusted for maternal age, race or ethnic group, and parity. [b] Included perinatal death, shoulder dystocia, bone fracture, and nerve palsy. [c]Defined as a birth weight of 4kg or greater.

- In a subgroup analysis of patients who completed quality of life (QOL) surveys, those in the intervention group had similar or higher QOL scores than the routine care group, suggesting that receiving a diagnosis of gestational diabetes did not diminish QOL.

Criticisms and Limitations:

- This study used the World Health Organization definition of gestational diabetes, which expanded in 1998 from patients with an intermediate glycemic response to any glycemic response above normal, including patients with a "diabetic" response. Women with severe glycemic intolerance, defined here as a glycemic response <198mg/dl (diabetic range) were not included; thus, the findings of the ACHOIS trial cannot be generalized to this patient population.
- This study population was recruited over the course of 10 years, spanning from 1993 to 2003. By the early 2000s, the use of oral agents for gestational diabetes management was being introduced with early studies suggesting favorable outcomes. The ACHOIS was not designed to study this emerging shift in treatment.
- Racial and ethnic groups studied were largely homogenous with White woman comprising ~75% of the study population, raising questions about generalizability of the study across ethnic groups as the dynamics of gestational diabetes is known to be different in different racial populations, country of origin, and so on.
- The median body mass index of the study for the intervention and routine care groups was 26.8 and 26, respectively; it may be difficult to generalize these findings to an obese patient population.

Other Relevant Studies and Information:

- The results from several other randomized control trials have further established that glycemic control of woman with mild carbohydrate intolerance in pregnancy results in a decrease in the rate of shoulder dystocia,[2,3] preeclampsia,[2,3] and birthweight greater than 4000g.[2-5]
- The Hyperglycemia and Adverse Pregnancy Outcomes (HAPO) study found greater risk with higher maternal glucose levels for adverse pregnancy outcomes such as premature delivery, shoulder dystocia, birth injury, and preeclampsia.[6]

Summary and Implications: The ACHOIS study is one of the first randomized control trials to investigate whether management of gestational diabetes can improve perinatal outcomes. The trial found that treating gestational diabetes is associated with improved maternal and fetal outcomes including decrease in macrosomia, birth trauma, shoulder dystocia, and preeclampsia. This and subsequent studies have shaped current ACOG guidelines, which recommend diet modification, glucose monitoring, and, if necessary, pharmacologic management for glycemic control in patients with gestational diabetes.[7] Insulin is considered the preferred treatment over oral medications.

CLINICAL CASE: MANAGEMENT OF GESTATIONAL DIABETES

Case History

A 26-year-old G2P1001 at 27 weeks and 4 days with history of normal spontaneous vaginal delivery presents for the routine prenatal visit. Her oral glucose tolerance test done prior to this visit suggests a diagnosis of gestational diabetes. Based on the ACHOIS study, what are your next steps in management?

Suggested Answer

The ACHOIS and subsequent studies demonstrated improved fetal and maternal outcomes in women with gestational diabetes with frequent blood sugar monitoring, proactive diet and exercise management, and initiation of pharmacologic management should glucose levels continue to be elevated. Patients should be counseled about the risks of uncontrolled glucose, particularly the increased risks of preeclampsia, shoulder dystocia, and macrosomia.

References

1. Crowther CA, Hiller JE, Moss JR, et al. Effect of treatment of gestational diabetes mellitus on pregnancy outcomes. *N Engl J Med.* 2005;352(24):2477–2486. doi:10.1056/NEJMoa042973
2. Bevier WC, Fishcer R, Jovanovic L. Treatment of women with an abnormal glucose challenge test (but a normal oral glucose tolerance test) decreases the risk of macrosomia. *Am J Perinatol.* 1999;16:269–275.
3. Landon MB, Spong CY, Thom E, Carpenter MW, Ramin SM, Casey B, et al., Eunice Kennedy Shriver National Institute of Child Health and Human Development Maternal-Fetal Medicine Units Network. A multicenter, randomized trial of treatment for mild gestational diabetes. *N Engl J Med.* 2009;361:1339–1348.

4. Bonomo M, Corica D, Mion E, Goncalves D, Motta G, Merati R, et al. Evaluating the therapeutic approach in pregnancies complicated by borderline: glucose intolerance: a randomized clinical trial. *Diabet Med.* 2005;22:1536–1541.

5. Garner P, Okun N, Keely E, Wells G, Perkins S, Sylvain J, et al. A randomized controlled trial of strict glycemic control and tertiary level obstetric care versus routine obstetric care in the management of gestational diabetes: a pilot study. *Am J Obstet Gynecol.* 1997;177:190–195.

6. HAPO Study Cooperative Research Group. Metzger BE, Lowe LP, Dyer AR, Trimble ER, Chaovarindr U, Coustan DR, Hadden DR, McCance DR, Hod M, McIntyre HD, Oats JJ, Persson B, Rogers MS, Sacks DA. Hyperglycemia and adverse pregnancy outcomes. *N Engl J Med.* 2008 May 8;358(19):1991–2002.

7. ACOG Practice Bulletin No. 190 Summary: gestational diabetes mellitus. *Obstet Gynecol.* 2018;131(2):406–408.

Reduction of Maternal–Infant Transmission of HIV Type 1 With Zidovudine Treatment

ELIZA RODRIGUE MCELWEE AND POOJA K. MEHTA

"Our study indicates that substantial reduction in the rate of maternal–infant transmission of HIV is possible with minimal short-term toxicity to mother or child."
— PEDIATRIC AIDS CLINICAL TRIALS PROTOCOL 76 STUDY GROUP[1]

Research Question: Does administration of antepartum, intrapartum, and neonatal zidovudine safely and effectively reduce the risk of maternal–infant human immunodeficiency virus type 1 (HIV-1) transmission?

Funding: The trial was supported by the National Institute of Allergy and Infectious Diseases, the National Institute of Child Health and Human Development, the Burroughs Wellcome Company in and the Agence Nationale de Recherche sur le SIDA

Year Study Began: 1991

Year Study Published: 1994

Study Location: 59 centers in France and the United States

Who Was Studied: HIV-infected pregnant women between 14 and 34 weeks gestational age who had a CD4+ T-lymphocyte count above 200 cells per cubic millimeter and had no existing indication for antiretroviral therapy.

Who Was Excluded: Pregnant women who demonstrated specific lab abnormalities (anemia, neutropenia, thrombocytopenia, renal impairment, or abnormal liver function); had received any antiretroviral treatment during the pregnancy; had previously received immunotherapy, anti-HIV vaccines, chemotherapeutic agents, or radiation therapy; had pregnancies with life-threatening anomalies oligohydramnios in the second trimester; had unexplained polyhydramnios in the third trimester; had evidence of fetal anemia; or had conditions that could increase fetal concentration of zidovudine or its metabolites.

How Many Patients: 477

Study Overview: This randomized, double-blind, placebo-controlled trial was discontinued at the first interim analysis, which showed that a three-part zidovudine regimen was effective in reducing HIV vertical transmission. See Figure 5.1

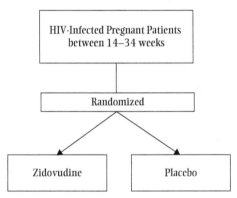

Figure 5.1. Study overview; the Pediatric AIDS Clinical Trial Group Protocol 76 Study Group

Study Intervention: Participants were stratified by gestational age. In the zidovudine arm, mothers received a standardized regimen of oral zidovudine antepartum (100mg 5 times daily) during pregnancy and a weight-based continuous intravenous (IV) zidovudine administration intrapartum. Infants born to mothers in this arm received a weight-based regimen of zidovudine for the first 6 weeks of life. Participants and their infants in the placebo arm did not receive antiviral treatment.

Follow-Up: Participants were monitored every 4 weeks until 32 weeks gestation, and then every 4 weeks until delivery. Sonograms were obtained before study entry and every 4 weeks after 28 weeks gestation. Women were seen 6 weeks and 6 months after delivery. Infants were followed through 18 months of life.

Endpoints: Primary outcome: Percentage HIV-infected infants at 18 months. Secondary outcomes: Maternal and infant adverse events (e.g., fetal or neonatal death) and toxic effects (e.g., anemia, neutropenia, thrombocytopenia, serum electrolyte abnormalities).

RESULTS

- The median gestational age of the live-born infants was 39 weeks; women received the study drug for a median of 11 weeks before giving birth. (See Table 5.1.)
- There was a 67.5% relative reduction in HIV transmission risk from mother to child in the zidovudine group ($p = 0.00006$). The study was discontinued early as this result crossed the predetermined interim analysis stopping p-value of 0.005.
- An increase in CD4+ lymphocyte values was observed in both study groups but was greater in the zidovudine group (141 vs. 101 cells per cubic millimeter, $p = 0.02$).
- The hemoglobin concentration at birth of infants in the zidovudine group was significantly lower than placebo, with maximal difference at 3 weeks of age and no difference by 12 weeks of age. Zidovudine treatment was not associated with neonatal death, premature birth, fetal growth, or structural abnormalities.
- The majority of maternal adverse effects that were reported were determined to be associated with obstetric complications and occurred in both placebo and intervention groups.

Table 5.1. KEY STUDY FINDINGS

	Zidovudine $n = 180$	Placebo $n = 183$
HIV infected	13	40
Probability of maternal–fetal HIV transmission at 18 months[a]	8.3%	25.5%

[a]Calculated by Kaplan-Meier method.

Criticisms and Limitations: Women were enrolled after the first trimester to avoid potential impact on fetal organogenesis, due to lack of safety data. This limited early exposure to zidovudine and may have impacted the rate of HIV transmission. Furthermore, treatment efficacy may be different in women with more advanced HIV disease, who may have increased viral load or zidovudine resistance. HIV initial viral load and viral load response were not assessed in this study; it is now widely acknowledged that viral load significantly impacts vertical transmission risk.

A debate emerged after the publication of this trial about the ethics of short-course zidovudine trials and withholding treatment from pregnant participants in the placebo arm.

Other Relevant Studies and Information:

- Further studies have since confirmed greater efficacy of *combination* antiretroviral therapy compared to zidovudine when administered antepartum to pregnant women (regardless of CD4+ T lymphocyte count and HIV viral load),[2] and with postpartum administration to infants.[3] Combination treatment regimens, however, are associated with a higher risk for neonatal and maternal adverse outcomes, including low birth weight and elevation in maternal liver enzymes.[4]
- The French Perinatal Cohort[5] evaluated HIV mother-to-child transmission in more than 11,000 HIV-positive pregnant women. The study demonstrated no significant reduction in HIV transmission with the administration of intrapartum zidovudine in the setting of a low HIV viral load (HIV RNA <1,000 copies/mL). This study suggests intrapartum antiretroviral therapy is not necessary for preventing vertical transmission in pregnant women with low viral load and further emphasizes the benefit of intrapartum therapy in the setting of higher viral loads.
- Current US treatment guidelines recommend that IV zidovudine should be administered to women with HIV RNA >1,000 copies/mL near delivery (or unknown HIV RNA levels), regardless of antepartum regimen. Antiretroviral therapy is not necessary for women receiving antiviral therapy with HIV RNA ≤1,000 copies/mL in late pregnancy and/or near delivery and for whom there are no concerns about adherence to or tolerance of their regimens but may be considered taking into account recent adherence, individual preferences, and provider judgement.[6]

Summary and Implications: This study demonstrated that a combination of antepartum, intrapartum, and neonatal antiretroviral therapy reduced perinatal transmission of HIV in women with mildly symptomatic disease and no prior antiretroviral treatment. This hallmark study is the stepping stone to additional work supporting the premise that antiretroviral therapy administered during pregnancy reduces risk of vertical transmission.[1]

CLINICAL CASE

A 27-year-old G2P1001 at 15 weeks gestational age with intrauterine pregnancy presents for antenatal care. She is newly diagnosed with HIV, with an elevated viral load of 2500 and CD4+ T-lymphocyte count of 235. She is concerned about HIV transmission to her infant. She asks about safety and efficacy of starting medication to help her and her baby at her current gestational age.

Suggested Answer

This study, as well as several others, demonstrates a significant decrease in vertical HIV transmission with the administration of antiretroviral therapy during the antepartum, intrapartum, and neonatal periods. Per current guidelines, a three-drug treatment regimen antepartum is recommended to reduce mother-to-child transmission, including intrapartum zidovudine administration as indicated based on viral load at the time of delivery.[6]

This theoretical patient has been newly diagnosed with HIV infection. She should be started on antiretroviral therapy at the earliest possible opportunity, which should be continued through delivery to decrease transmission of HIV to the child. Viral load should be reassessed at least once per trimester and again prior to delivery to inform decisions about intrapartum zidovudine administration and mode of delivery.

References

1. Connor EM, Sperling RS, Gelber R, et al. Reduction of maternal–infant transmission of human immunodeficiency virus type 1 with zidovudine treatment. Pediatric AIDS Clinical Trials Group Protocol 076 Study Group. *N Engl J Med.* 1994;331(18):1173–1180.
2. Cooper ER, Charurat M, Mofenson L, Hanson IC, Pitt J, Diaz C, Blattner W. Combination antiretroviral strategies for the treatment of pregnant HIV-1-infected women and prevention of perinatal HIV-1 transmission. *J Acquir Immune Defic Syndr.* 2002;29(5):484–494.

3. Nielsen-Saines K, Watts DH, Veloso VG, et al. Three postpartum anti-retroviral regimens to prevent intrapartum HIV infection. *N Engl J Med.* 2012;366(25):2368–2379.
4. Fowler MG, Qin M, Fiscus S, Currier J, et al. Benefits and risks of antiretroviral therapy for perinatal HIV prevention. *N Engl J Med.* 2016;375:1726–1737.
5. Briand N, Warszawski J, Mendelbrot L, et al. Is intrapartum intravenous Zidovudine for prevention of mother-to-child HIV-1 transmission still useful in the combination antiretroviral therapy era? *Clin Infect Dis.* 2013 Sep;57(6):903–914.
6. Panel on Treatment of Pregnant Women with HIV Infection and Prevention of Perinatal Transmission. Recommendations for the Use of Antiretroviral Drugs in Pregnant Women with HIV Infection and Interventions to Reduce Perinatal HIV Transmission in the United States. Available at http://aidsinfo.nih.gov/contentfiles/lvguidelines/PerinatalGL.pdf

6

The Length of the Cervix and the Risk
of Spontaneous Preterm Delivery

JULIE STONE AND MICHAEL HOUSE

"There is a continuum of cervical performance that is reflected function-
ally by the gestational age of the infant delivered prematurely and ana-
tomically by the length of the cervix."

—JD IAMS ET AL.[1]

Research Question: Is a short cervix associated with an increased risk of spontaneous preterm birth?

Funding: The Eunice Kennedy Shriver National Institute of Child Health and
Human Development

Year Study Began: 1992–1994

Year Study Published: 1996

Study Location: 10 university-affiliated prenatal clinics in the Maternal Fetal
Medicine Network of the National Institute of the Child Health and Human
Development.

Who Was Studied: Women with singleton pregnancies before 24 weeks' gestation were recruited.

Who Was Excluded: Patients with multiple gestation, cerclage, placenta previa, or a major fetal anomaly were excluded.

How Many Patients: 2,915

Study Overview: See Figure 6.1

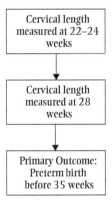

Figure 6.1 Study overview

Cervical length and funneling were evaluated as potential variables predictive of preterm delivery. All patients had a real-time transvaginal ultrasound performed with the bladder emptied between 22–24 6/7 weeks' gestation (24-week visit) and again 4 weeks later (28-week visit). Cervical length in centimeters was recorded. Also, the presence or absence of a funnel was recorded. A digital cervical exam preceded each ultrasound measurement, and the Bishop score was correlated with cervical length.

Follow-Up: The first study visit occurred between 22–24 6/7 weeks' gestation. Subsequent visits were at 2, 4, and 6 weeks afterwards.

Endpoints: The primary outcome was spontaneous preterm birth before 35 weeks' gestation. Spontaneous preterm birth was defined as preterm birth arising from preterm labor or preterm premature rupture of the membranes.

RESULTS

- The key finding of the study was that a short cervix is associated with subsequent preterm birth. The relative risk of preterm birth increased as cervical length decreased, see Table 6.1 and Figure 6.2.

Table 6.1. Relative Risk of Preterm Birth for Different
Cervical Length Cutoff Values

Short Cervix Length Cutoff (mm)	% of Women	Relative Risk of Spontaneous Preterm Birth[a] (95% Confidence Interval)
40	75	1.98 (1.2–3.3)
35	50	2.35 (1.4–3.9)
30	25	3.79 (2.3–6.2)
26	10	6.19 (3.8–10.0)
22	5	9.49 (6.0–15.2)
13	1	13.99 (7.9–24.8)

[a] Relative risk of preterm birth compared to women with cervical length over 40 mm (above the 75th percentile).

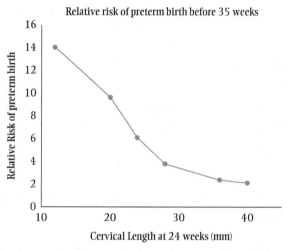

Figure 6.2 The relative risk of preterm birth as a function of cervical length. As cervical length decreases, the relative risk of preterm birth before 35 weeks increases, indicating an inverse relationship.

- There were small differences in cervical length between nulliparous and multiparous women, but the differences were clinically insignificant. Data for parous and nulliparous women were combined. The mean ± standard deviation cervical length at 24 weeks was 35.2 ± 8.3mm.
- Among parous women, the number of previous deliveries had no effect on the length of the cervix.
- Cervical shortening between 24 to 28 weeks was associated with a modest increase in preterm birth risk compared to no shortening (relative risk 2.03; 95% confidence interval 1.28–3.22).

- Receiver-operating-characteristic curves suggested cervical length less than 25mm as a threshold value for clinical use. When the cervix was less than 25mm at 24 weeks, the sensitivity, specificity, positive predictive value, and negative predictive value for predicting preterm birth before 35 weeks was 37.3%, 92.2%, 17.8%, and 97%, respectively.
- Funneling was a significant predictor of preterm birth even after controlling for cervical length. The data on funneling, however, showed substantial variation among study centers.

Criticisms and Limitations: The pathophysiology of cervical shortening is difficult to establish. Preterm birth is a syndrome caused by multiple causes.[2] Cervical shortening can be the final common pathway of cervical insufficiency, intrauterine infection/inflammation, and preterm labor. Although the study established the association of a short cervix and subsequent preterm birth, it did not determine the cause of cervical shortening.

Other Relevant Studies and Information:

- Subsequent studies established that a short cervix measured earlier in gestation (e.g., 16–18 weeks was associated with preterm birth).[3]
- Randomized trials used cervical shortening to target patients appropriate for therapy to prevent preterm birth. In the setting of a short cervix, both vaginal progesterone[4] and cerclage[5] have been evaluated as interventions that may prevent preterm birth.
- In current practice, measurement of cervical length is a central feature of the American College of Obstetricians and Gynecologists management protocol to prevent preterm birth.[6]
- When transabdominal imaging at the anatomy survey suggests a short cervix is present, it is recommended to perform a vaginal ultrasound for improved visualization of cervical length.[6]
- For women with a history of a spontaneous preterm birth, serial transvaginal cervical length screening is recommend from 16 to 23 weeks every 1 to 2 weeks.[6,7]

Summary and Implications: A short cervix is associated with increased preterm birth risk.

This study demonstrated an inverse relationship between cervical length and risk of preterm birth; the shortest cervix conferred the highest risk of preterm birth. Based on this and other studies, serial cervical length measurements are recommended for women with a history of spontaneous preterm birth and for women with a suspected short cervix on transabdominal ultrasound. If a short cervix is seen, vaginal progesterone and/or cervical cerclage may be considered to reduce the risk of preterm birth depending on the clinical situation.

CLINICAL CASE: THE LENGTH OF THE CERVIX AND THE RISK OF PRETERM BIRTH

Case History

A 32-year-old G3P0111 presents at 16 weeks for a new prenatal visit. She has a history of spontaneous vaginal delivery at 31 weeks for preterm labor with her first child. She has no significant medical or surgical history. She denies any cramping, vaginal bleeding, or leakage of fluid. Ultrasound confirms a viable 16-week intrauterine pregnancy.

What other measurement should be obtained?

Suggested Answer

The cervical length should be measured using a transvaginal ultrasound. If cervical length is less than 2.5 cm, cerclage can be offered. If cervical length is greater than 2.5 cm, serial measurements should be scheduled every 1 to 2 weeks until 23 weeks to assess for cervical shortening.[7]

References

1. Iams JD, Goldenberg RL, Meis PJ, Mercer BM, Moawad A, Das A, et al. The length of the cervix and the risk of spontaneous premature delivery. *N Engl J Med.* 1996;334:567.
2. Romero R, Dey SK, Fisher SJ. Preterm labor: one syndrome, many causes. *Science.* 2014;345:760.
3. Owen J, Yost N, Berghella V, Thom E, Swain M, Dildy GA, 3rd, et al. Mid-trimester endovaginal sonography in women at high risk for spontaneous preterm birth. *JAMA.* 2001;286:1340.
4. Fonseca EB, Celik E, Parra M, Singh M, Nicolaides KH, Fetal Medicine Foundation Second Trimester Screening Group. Progesterone and the risk of preterm birth among women with a short cervix. *N Engl J Med.* 2007;357:462.
5. Owen J, Hankins G, Iams JD, Berghella V, Sheffield JS, Perez-Delboy A, et al. Multicenter randomized trial of cerclage for preterm birth prevention in

high-risk women with shortened midtrimester cervical length. *Am J Obstet Gynecol.* 2009;201:375.

6. ACOG Practice Bulletin No. 130: prediction and prevention of preterm birth. *Obstet Gynecol.* 2012;120:964.

7. Iams JD, Berghella V. Care for women with prior preterm birth. *Am J Obstet Gynecol.* 2010;203:89.

Intramuscular Progesterone for the Prevention of Recurrent Preterm Birth

EMILY A. OLIVER AND AMANDA ROMAN-CAMARGO

"Weekly injections of 17P resulted in a substantial reduction in the rate of recurrent preterm delivery among women who were at particularly high risk for preterm delivery and reduced the likelihood of several complications in their infants."

—PJ MEIS ET AL.[1]

Research Question: Does 17 alpha-hydroxyprogesterone caproate (17P) prevent recurrent preterm delivery?[1]

Funding: National Institute of Child Health and Human Development

Year Study Began: 1998[a]

Year Study Published: 2003

Study Location: 19 participating centers in the United States

Who Was Included: Pregnant women between 16 and 20 weeks with a history of spontaneous preterm delivery (between 20 and 36 completed weeks).

---

[a] The study was started in 1998; data prior to 1999 was not included.

Who Was Excluded: Women whose pregnancies were complicated by a multifetal gestation; known fetal anomaly; who were on progesterone or heparin treatment; had a cervical cerclage in place or planned, chronic hypertension on medication, seizure disorder, or plans to deliver at another institution.

How Many Patients: 463

Study Overview: This was a randomized controlled trial. See Figure 7.1

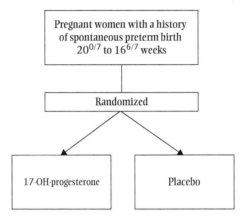

Figure 7.1. Study overview

Study Intervention: Participants were randomized to receive either 17P or an identically packaged placebo. Both the patients and providers were blinded to the group assignment. Study treatment was administered intramuscular and weekly, from 16 weeks up to 36 weeks of gestation. The women continued to receive standard prenatal care.

Follow-Up: Women were followed until delivery, infants were followed until discharge either from the hospital in which the birth occurred, or if they were transferred, from the hospital to which they were transferred.

Endpoints: The primary outcome was preterm birth, defined as delivery before 37 weeks of gestation. Secondary outcomes included: miscarriage, stillbirth, infant outcomes including birthweight less than 2500g, necrotizing enterocolitis, need for supplemental oxygen, intraventricular hemorrhage, infant death.

RESULTS

- Frequency of preterm delivery (<37 weeks) was 36.3% in the progesterone group versus 54.9% in the placebo group (p <0.001).
- The frequency of delivery before 35 weeks was 20.6% in the progesterone group versus 30.7% in the placebo group (p = 0.02). The difference in deliveries before 32 weeks was also statistically significant (11.4% vs. 19.6%, p = 0.02).
- After adjusting for the number of prior preterm births, the relative risk of preterm birth was 0.70 (95% confidence interval (CI); 0.57–0.85) in the progesterone group.
- There were no statistically significant differences in the rate of miscarriages and stillbirths.
- There was a significant decrease in birthweight less than 2500g (relative risk (RR) 0.66, 95% CI: 0.51–0.87) and need for supplemental oxygen (RR 0.62, 95% CI 0.42–0.92) in the progesterone group. There were no significant differences in the other neonatal outcomes. (See Table 7.1.)

Table 7.1. PREGNANCY OUTCOMES ACCORDING TO RANDOMIZATION

	Progesterone Group (%)	Placebo Group (%)	Relative Risk (95% Confidence Interval)
Preterm delivery before 37 weeks	36.3	54.9	0.66 (0.54–0.81)
Preterm delivery before 35 weeks	20.6	30.7	0.67 (0.48–0.93)
Preterm delivery before 32 weeks	11.4	19.6	0.58 (0.37–0.91)
Birth weight <2500g	27.2	41.1	0.66 (0.51–0.87)
Birth weight <1500g	8.6.	14.6	0.62 (0.36–1.07)
Neonatal death	2.6	5.9	0.44 (0.17–1.13)

Criticisms and Limitations: This study included women with a particularly high incidence of preterm birth, with 54.9% in the placebo controlled group having a recurrent preterm delivery. The mean gestational age of the prior preterm birth was 31 weeks, and half the women had a history of 2 or more preterm births. The ability to extrapolate these results to other populations remains unknown.

Other Relevant Studies and Information:

- Several trials of women with a history of prior preterm birth have also demonstrated a significant reduction in preterm birth <37 weeks and perinatal mortality with 17P 250 mg IM weekly compared to placebo.[2,5]
- Vaginal progesterone has also been studied and generally been demonstrated to perform more poorly or, at best, no better than 17P.[3,4,6]
- In 2019 the PROLONG trial (17OHPC to Prevent Recurrent Preterm Birth in Singleton Gestations) concluded, contrary to Meis et al., that patients taking 17P did not have a reduction in preterm birth or neonatal morbidity. The Meis et al. study differed from the PROLONG trial in that (a) the incidence of recurrent preterm birth in the placebo arm was more than 2 times that of the PROLONG study, and (b) the racial breakdown of the study population was much more homogenous, with <10% enrollees identified as Black in the PROLONG trial.[7]
- ACOG and SMFM guidelines currently recommend 17P to be given weekly starting between 16 to 20 weeks until 36 weeks for women with a history of spontaneous preterm birth.[8]

Summary and Implications: In women with a history of spontaneous preterm birth, weekly intramuscular 17P, starting between 16 and 20 weeks though 36 weeks' gestation, decreases the rate of recurrent preterm birth prior to 37 weeks compared to placebo.

CLINICAL CASE

Case History

A 23-year-old G1P0101 had an uncomplicated pregnancy until around 32 weeks. She presented with back pain and contractions and was found to be 2cm dilated. Shortly after presenting she ruptured her membranes, her contractions worsened and she had a spontaneous preterm vaginal delivery.

The patient returns postpartum and would like to discuss how her next pregnancy would be managed. Based on the results of this trial, how would you advise this patient?

Suggested Answer

This trial showed that in women with a history of spontaneous preterm birth, administering 17P intramuscularly weekly from 16 weeks' gestational age until 36 weeks decreased the risk of preterm birth. Therefore, she should be offered treatment with weekly 17P starting at 16 weeks until 36 weeks.

References

1. Meis PJ, Klebanoff M, Thom E, et al. Prevention of recurrent preterm delivery by 17 alpha-hydroxyprogesterone caproate. *N Engl J Med.* 2003;348(24):2379–2385.
2. Johnson JW, Austin KL, Jones GS, Davis GH, King TM. Efficacy of 17 alpha-hydroxyprogesterone caproate in the prevention of premature labor. *N Engl J Med.* 1975;293(14):675–680.
3. da Fonseca EB, Bittar RE, Carvalho MH, Zugaib M. Prophylactic administration of progesterone by vaginal suppository to reduce the incidence of spontaneous preterm birth in women at increased risk: a randomized placebo-controlled double-blind study. *Am J Obstet Gynecol.* 2003;188(2):419–424.
4. O'Brien JM, Adair CD, Lewis DF, et al. Progesterone vaginal gel for the reduction of recurrent preterm birth: primary results from a randomized, double-blind, placebo-controlled trial. *Ultrasound Obstet Gynecol.* 2007;30(5):687–696.
5. Maher MA, Abdelaziz A, Ellaithy M, Bazeed MF. Prevention of preterm birth: a randomized trial of vaginal compared with intramuscular progesterone. *Acta Obstet Gynecol Scand.* 2013;92(2):215–222.
6. El-Gharib MN, El-Hawary. Matched sample comparison of intramuscular versus vaginal micronized progesterone for prevention of preterm birth. *J Matern Fetal Neonatal Med.* 2013;26(7):716–719.
7. Blackwell SC, Gyamfi-Bannerman C, Biggio JR Jr, et al. 17-OHPC to Prevent Recurrent Preterm Birth in Singleton Gestations (PROLONG Study): a multicenter, international, randomized double-blind trial. *Am J Perinatol.* 2020;37(2):127–136.
8. Society of Maternal-Fetal Medicine. Progesterone and preterm birth prevention: translating clinical trials data into clinical practice. *Am J Obstet Gynecol.* 2012 May;206(5):376–386.

8

Antibiotics for Preterm Premature Rupture of Membranes

KATHERINE S. KOHARI AND CHRISTIAN M. PETTKER

"Antibiotic treatment of expectantly managed women with PPROM . . .
will reduce infectious and gestational age-dependent infant morbidity."
—BM MERCER ET AL.[1]

Research Question: Should patient's presenting with preterm prelabor rupture of membranes (PPROM) be given antibiotics to improve perinatal morbidity and mortality?

Funding: National Institute of Child Health and Human Development Maternal-Fetal Medicine Units Network

Year Study Began: 1992

Year Study Published: 1997

Study Location: 11 clinical centers in the United States

Who Was Studied: Pregnant women between 24 weeks and 32 weeks presenting with PPROM who were being considered for expectant management.

Who Was Excluded: Patients with fever requiring antibiotics, recent antibiotic and/or corticosteroid use, allergies to penicillin and/or erythromycin, significant medical conditions, placenta previa, vaginal bleeding, indication for delivery, estimated fetal weight below 10th percentile, and fetal malformations were excluded.

How Many Patients: 614

Study Overview: This was a randomized controlled trial. See Figure 8.1

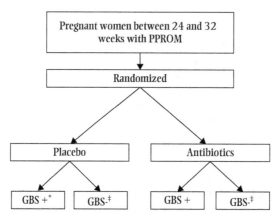

Figure 8.1. Study overview
*GBS positive patients in the placebo/control group received a 1-week course of ampicillin.
†Primary analysis additionally performed on GBS—groups to avoid confounding with antibiotic treatment of GBS.

Study Intervention: Patients in the antibiotic group received ampicillin 2gm intravenous (IV) every 6 hours and erythromycin 250mg IV every 8 hours for 48 hours followed by amoxicillin 250mg orally every 8 hours and erythromycin 333mg orally every 8 hours for 5 days. The placebo group received visually indistinguishable IV and oral regimens. Women who tested positive for Group B streptococcus (GBS), even those in the control group, were treated a 7-day course of oral ampicillin and IV ampicillin in labor.

Patients were managed inpatient and monitored with daily clinical assessment for signs of infection, as well as daily fetal nonstress testing. Antenatal corticosteroids and tocolysis were not permitted after enrollment. Elective delivery was prohibited prior to 34 weeks and expectant management discouraged after 34 weeks.

Follow-Up: Patients were followed concurrently. Neonates were followed until discharge or death.

Primary outcome: Composite neonatal outcome including fetal/infant death, neonatal respiratory distress, severe intraventricular hemorrhage, stage 2 or 3 necrotizing enterocolitis, or sepsis (<72 hours).

Secondary outcome: Investigators evaluated other infant morbidities, maternal outcomes, pregnancy outcomes, and adverse effects of and compliance with the regimen.

RESULTS

- The primary analysis was performed in the GBS negative cohort. Composite morbidity was significantly lower in the GBS negative cohort that was randomized to receive antibiotics (44.5% vs. 54.5%, $p=0.03$). There was no decrease in morbidity in the GBS positive cohort. (See Table 8.1.)
- GBS negative patients who received antibiotics generally remained pregnant significantly longer (median of 6.1 days vs. 2.9 days to delivery, $p <0.001$). A greater proportion of these patients receiving antibiotics remained pregnant each day than of those who did not.
- Rates of neonatal respiratory distress were significantly lower in the antibiotic group (40.8% vs. 50.6%), although the rates of each of the component morbidities that made up the composite outcome were similar in the GBS negative group.
- Antibiotic therapy was associated with reduced rates of patent ductus arteriosus and bronchopulmonary dysplasia in the entire cohort. There were no differences in rates of neonatal sepsis or pneumonia in the entire cohort, though there was a reduction in neonatal sepsis after 72 hours and pneumonia in the GBS negative cohort.

Table 8.1. OUTCOMES IN ALL PATIENTS

Outcome	Antibiotic Group (%) $n = 299$	Placebo (%) $n = 312$	p-value	Relative Risk (95% Confidence Interval)
Composite Morbidity	44.1	52.9	.04	0.84 (0.71–0.99)
Respiratory Distress	40.5	48.7	.04	0.83 (0.69–0.99)
NEC stage II or III	2.3	5.8	.03	0.84 (0.71–0.99)
>1 Outcome	12.4	16.0	.19	0.77 (0.51–1.15)

Criticisms and Limitations: The study prohibited the administration of antenatal corticosteroids for fetal lung maturity. While this allowed for reduction in possible confounding with steroid exposure, lack of corticosteroid exposure makes these results less generalizable, as it is now considered the standard of care for patients with PPROM.

Furthermore, patients were enrolled only until 32 weeks and 0 days while planned delivery did not occur until 34 weeks, leaving a temporal gap of patients in which these results do not apply. The patient population is comprised of mainly women of color (>70%) and those receiving government assistance (>75%) being treated in an academic setting and therefore may not be generalizable to all patient populations.

Other Relevant Studies and Information:

- This trial was one of the first large-scale randomized controlled trials to demonstrate prolonged latency and improved neonatal outcomes with antibiotic treatment for PPROM.
- A 2013 Cochrane systematic review of 22 trials supports the initial findings of Mercer et al. pertaining to prolonged latency and reduced neonatal morbidity.[2]
- Several antibiotic regimens have been evaluated with similar efficacy. These regimens include coverage for major pelvic pathogens such as Group B *Streptococcus, Ureaplasma,* anaerobes, and *Chlamydia trachomatis.*[3,4]
- The "Mercer Protocol" is considered the standard of care, but several alternate regimens are recognized as acceptable alternatives. Regimens have evolved over the years, especially in the face of a shortage of IV erythromycin. Some centers use azithromycin (such as a single oral dose of azithromycin 1g) when erythromycin is not available or if tolerance is an issue.[3]
- Guidelines set forth by the American College of Obstetricians and Gynecologists recommend initiation of broad spectrum antibiotics in the setting of PPROM when <34 weeks.[5]

Summary and Implications: This trial demonstrated the benefits of broad spectrum antibiotics for women presenting with PPROM. The Mercer Protocol, as this regimen is often referred to, is now the standard of care for all patients with viable pregnancies less than 34 weeks of gestation. Based on this and other studies, antibiotic therapy is now recommended for all women presenting with PPROM at less than 34 weeks of gestation to prolong latency and improve neonatal outcomes.[5]

CLINICAL CASE: ANTIBIOTICS FOR PRETERM PRELABOR RUPTURE OF MEMBRANES

Case History

A 23-year-old G1P0010 presents to Labor and Delivery at 27 weeks and 5 days of gestation with the complaint of leakage of fluid. Her prenatal course has otherwise been uncomplicated. On examination, she is noted to have copious amounts of amniotic fluid coming from a closed cervical os. Based upon the findings of this research, what is the next best step in management of this patient?

Suggested Answer

The patient presents with PPROM. Based on the findings of Mercer et al., administration of broad-spectrum antibiotics for patients with PPROM, results in improved clinical outcomes due to prolonged latency of pregnancy. Patients should receive a workup for comorbid infection, including GBS, chlamydia/gonorrhea, and urine culture. The Mercer Protocol is as follows: administration of IV erythromycin and ampicillin, followed by PO erythromycin and amoxicillin, although other regimens have demonstrated equivalent efficacy. Current guidelines call for administration of betamethasone to promote fetal lung maturity and, at <32 weeks of gestation, magnesium sulfate for fetal neuroprotection. Delivery is indicated at 34 weeks, or earlier with labor or signs/symptoms of infection.

References

1. Mercer BM, Miodovnik M, Thurnau GR, et al. Antibiotic therapy for reduction of infant morbidity after preterm premature rupture of the membranes: a randomized controlled trial. *JAMA.* 1997;278(12): 989–995.
2. Kenyon S, et al. Antibiotics for preterm rupture of membranes. *Cochrane Database Syst Rev.* 2013.
3. Pierson RC, Gordon SS, Haas DM. A retrospective comparison of antibiotic regimens for preterm premature rupture of membranes. *Obstet Gynecol.* 2014;124(3):515–519.
4. Lee J, Romero R, Kim SM, et al. A new antibiotic regimen treats and prevents intra-amniotic inflammation/infection in patients with preterm PROM. *J Matern Fetal Neonatal Med.* 2016;29(17):2727–2737.
5. ACOG Practice Bulletin Number 188. Prelabor Rupture of Membranes, January 2018.

9

Fetal Fibronectin in Cervical and Vaginal Secretions as a Predictor of Preterm Delivery

ZACHARY COLVIN AND ANNA PALATNIK

"The release of fibronectin bearing the oncofetal domain into the cervicovaginal secretions of pregnant women during the second and third trimesters can be used to distinguish between symptomatic patients who will deliver prematurely and those who will deliver at term."

—CJ LOCKWOOD ET AL.[1]

Research Question: Is the presence of fetal fibronectin in the cervical and vaginal secretions of pregnant women correlated with their risk for preterm delivery?

Funding: The Kennedy-Dannreuther Fellowship from the American Association of Obstetricians and Gynecologists Foundation, Revson Foundation, and Adeza Biomedical.

Year Study Published: 1991

Study Location: Mount Sinai Medical Center, New York, New York; St. Margaret's Hospital, Boston, Massachusetts; University of California at Irvine, Irvine, California.

Who Was Studied: Study patients were pregnant women with precise gestational dating evaluated for either preterm premature rupture of membranes (PPROM) or preterm contractions with intact membranes. Control patients were pregnant women without complications of preterm contractions, vaginal bleeding, or PPROM.

Who Was Excluded: Women whose pregnancy was complicated by presence of congenital anomalies, placenta previa, intercourse within the last 24 hours of examination, or previous pregnancies terminated before term because of maternal hypertension, fetal growth restriction, or fetal distress.

How Many Patients: 345

Study Overview: See Figure 9.1 for a summary of the study design.

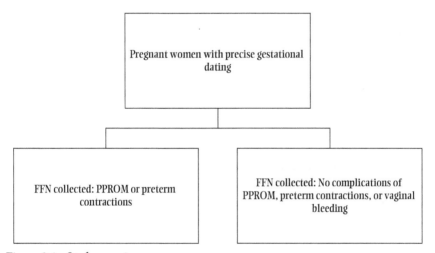

Figure 9.1. Study overview

Study Intervention: After meeting eligibility criteria, the study patients underwent a sterile speculum exam where samples of both the cervical and posterior vaginal forniceal mucus were collected and tested for fetal fibronectin concentration. Control patients had samples of cervical and vaginal mucus taken and assayed for fetal fibronectin an average of 4 times between 5 and 40 weeks' gestation. Concentrations of fetal fibronectin antigen were measured with a sensitive immunoassay that uses a fetal fibronectin-specific monoclonal antibody FDC-6.

Follow-Up: Study and control patients were followed until delivery.

Endpoints: Preterm delivery <37 weeks

RESULTS

- Fetal fibronectin was demonstrated to have a sensitivity of 81.7% and a specificity of 82.5% for preterm delivery based on the results of this study. See Table 9.1.
- Women with uncomplicated pregnancies who delivered at term had only 4% of cervical and 3% of vaginal samples positive for fetal fibronectin between 21 and 37 weeks.
- There were significantly more samples positive for fetal fibronectin in this uncomplicated population prior to 22 weeks and after 37 weeks.
- Among women with PPROM, 93.8% of the cervicovaginal samples were positive for fetal fibronectin.
- Women with preterm contractions who had a positive cervical or vaginal sample for fetal fibronectin were more likely to deliver preterm than those with negative samples (83.1% vs. 19.0%, p <0.01).
- Significant independent predictors of preterm delivery were cervicovaginal fetal fibronectin, cervical dilation, and tocolytic therapy.

Table 9.1. FETAL FIBRONECTIN TEST RESULTS AND OUTCOMES IN PATIENTS WITH PRETERM UTERINE CONTRACTIONS

Fetal Fibronectin	Pregnancy Outcome		Total Number of Patients	
	Number Patients with Preterm Delivery (<37 weeks)	Number of Patients with Term Delivery (≥ 37 weeks)		
Present	49	10	59	Positive predictive value = 83.1%
Negative	11	47	58	Negative predictive value = 81.0%
Total	60	57	117	
	Sensitivity = 81.7%	Specificity = 82.5%		

Criticisms and Limitations: The study included women with various cervical dilations; raising the question that fetal fibronectin positivity could be affected by cervical dilation and possibly confounding the results. Fetal fibronectin's best predictive value is among women with minimal cervical dilation.

Other Relevant Studies and Information:

- Studies published subsequent to this have also reported increased risk of preterm birth with positive fetal fibronectin among women symptomatic for labor.[2–4]
- A multicenter trial by Peaceman et al.[5] showed a negative predictive value of 99.5% for delivery within 7 days. There was no clinical advantage with routine testing for fetal fibronectin.
- A 2016 meta-analysis by Berghella et al.[6] of 6 randomized clinical trials showed that fetal fibronectin testing among women with threatened preterm labor was not associated with prevention of preterm birth or improvement in perinatal outcomes and was associated with higher costs.
- A few studies evaluated the predictive power of fetal fibronectin testing combined with cervical length in symptomatic women.[6,7] Their results suggest that the combination may improve prediction of spontaneous preterm birth management in women with cervical length 15 to 30mm.
- A large, multicenter trial by Esplin et al.[8] showed that quantitative vaginal fetal fibronectin and serial transvaginal ultrasound cervical lengths have low predictive accuracy as a screening test in predicting preterm birth among nulliparous women with singleton pregnancies. In this study, the negative predictive value of a negative result (< 50ng/ml) was 95.7%.
- The American College of Obstetricians and Gynecologists and the Society for Maternal-Fetal Medicine do not recommend fetal fibronectin as a screening test to assess for risk of preterm birth among asymptomatic women. Fetal fibronectin screening is suggested as a possible tool in managing symptomatic women with suspected preterm labor at or before 34 weeks.[9,10]

Summary and Implications: This study demonstrated that the presence of cervical or vaginal fetal fibronectin may help identify those at increased risk of preterm delivery among women with preterm contractions and intact membranes.

CLINICAL CASE: FETAL FIBRONECTIN AS A PREDICTOR OF PRETERM DELIVERY

Case History

A 27-year-old G2P1001 at 29 weeks of gestation presents to the hospital with abdominal cramping. Her pregnancy was uncomplicated and she has no pertinent past medical history. She had regular, symptomatic uterine contractions every 2 to 4 minutes. Her cervix was 1 cm dilated, 50% effaced,—3 station with intact membranes. She was given intravenous fluids and reexamined 2 hours later. Cervical exam was unchanged, but the patient continued to have regular contractions. A fetal fibronectin swab was collected on admission prior to the first cervical exam and was negative. How can these results be used to help manage the patient?

Suggested Answer

The presence of cervical or vaginal fetal fibronectin can help identify those at increased risk of preterm delivery in patients with preterm contractions with intact membranes. Alternatively, the absence of cervical or vaginal fetal fibronectin can reasonably predict those who will not deliver in the next 7 to 14 days with a high negative predictive value. In our patient, who has no risk factors for preterm delivery except preterm contractions, negative fetal fibronectin can help reassure both the patient and her provider to withhold further medical interventions (corticosteroids, magnesium sulfate, tocolytics, antibiotics) and discharge the patient home after a period of observation. Outpatient follow-up may be scheduled in 1 week.

In contrast, if fetal fibronectin test came back positive, the decision regarding initiation of interventions to reduce morbidity associated with preterm delivery should be guided by the entire clinical scenario. The positive predictive value of positive fetal fibronectin is low, and thus it should not by itself guide patient management. In that case, a few management options are reasonable: (a) continue in-patient observation with serial digital cervical exams and begin medical interventions if cervix continues to dilate or efface; (b) measure cervical length and, if it is shortened (<25mm–30mm), then begin medical interventions; (c) begin medical interventions without performing cervical length, based on clinical risk factors.

References

1. Lockwood CJ, et al. Fetal fibronectin in cervical and vaginal secretions as a predictor of preterm delivery. *NEJM*. 1991;325(10):669–674.
2. Peaceman AM, et al. Fetal fibronectin as a predictor of preterm birth in patients with symptoms: a multicenter trial. *Am J Obstet Gynecol*. 1997;177(1):13–18.
3. Skoll A, et al. The evaluation of the fetal fibronectin test for prediction of preterm delivery in symptomatic patients. *J Obstet Gynaecol Can*. 2006;28(3):206–213.
4. Swamy GK, et al. Clinical utility of fetal fibronectin for predicting preterm birth. *J Reprod Med* 2005;50(11):851–856.
5. Berghella V, et al. Fetal fibronectin testing for prevention of preterm birth in singleton pregnancies with threatened preterm labor: a systematic review and metaanalysis of randomized controlled trials. *Am J Obstet Gynecol*. 2016;215(4):431–438.
6. Gomez R, et al. Cervicovaginal fibronectin improves the prediction of preterm delivery based on sonographic cervical length in patients with preterm uterine contractions and intact membranes. *Am J Obstet Gynecol*. 2005;192 (2):350–359.
7. Van Baaren GJ, et al. Predictive value of cervical length measurement and fibronectin testing in threatened preterm labor. *Obstet Gynecol*. 2014;123(6):1185–1192.
8. Esplin MS, Elovitz MA, Iams JD, et al. Predictive accuracy of serial transvaginal cervical lengths and quantitative vaginal fetal fibronectin levels for spontaneous preterm birth among nulliparous women. *JAMA*. 2017;317(10):1047–1056.
9. Prediction and prevention of preterm birth. Practice Bulletin No. 130. American College of Obstetricians and Gynecologists. *Obstet Gynecol*. 2012;120: 964–973.
10. Progesterone and preterm birth prevention: translating clinical trials data into clinical practice. *Am J Obstet Gynecol*. 2012;206(5):376–386.

Magnesium Sulfate for the Prevention of Cerebral Palsy

The BEAM Trial

LAURA SMITH AND BLAIR J. WYLIE

"Our findings suggest that magnesium sulfate may reduce the chance that cerebral palsy will subsequently be diagnosed in a child who was at high risk for preterm birth."

—THE BEAM INVESTIGATORS[1]

Research Question: Does administration of magnesium sulfate to women at risk for preterm birth reduce the risk of cerebral palsy?

Funding: The National Institute of Child Health and Human Development and the National Institute of Neurological Disorders and Stroke

Year Study Began: 1997 (enrollment completed in May 2004)

Year Study Published: 2008

Study Location: 20 predominantly academic medical centers across the United States participating in the Eunice Kennedy Shriver National Institute of Child Health and Human Development Maternal-Fetal Medicine Units (MFMU) Network

Who Was Studied: Women carrying live singleton or twin gestations at high risk for imminent preterm birth between 24 and 31 6/7 weeks' gestation with at least one of the following indications:

- premature rupture of membranes
- advanced preterm labor defined as cervical dilation of 4 to 8 cm
- indicated preterm birth planned within 2 to 24 hours

Who Was Excluded: Patients with anticipated delivery within 2 hours, cervical dilation greater than 8cm, rupture of membranes occurring at less than 22 weeks, fetal anomalies if the obstetrics team was unwilling to intervene on behalf of fetus, or if fetal demise occurred prior to enrollment. Patients with comorbid maternal hypertension or preeclampsia, contraindications to magnesium sulfate, or receipt of magnesium sulfate within prior 12 hours (e.g., as in use for tocolysis) were also excluded.

How Many Patients: 2,241

Study Overview: This was a randomized controlled trial. See Figure 10.1

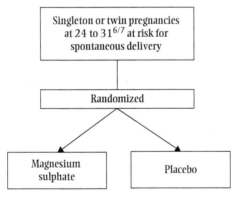

Figure 10.1. Study overview

Study Intervention: Patients were randomized to receive either magnesium sulfate or placebo. The magnesium sulfate protocol included a 6g initial bolus followed by a 2g maintenance infusion. The infusion (magnesium or placebo) was stopped if delivery had not occurred within 12 hours but resumed if delivery was thought to again be imminent.

Follow-Up: Infants followed through 2 years of age, corrected for prematurity

Endpoints: Primary outcome: A composite outcome comprised of stillbirth, infant death by age 1, and moderate to severe cerebral palsy by age 2. Secondary outcomes: Individual outcomes of stillbirth, infant death by age 1, moderate to moderate/severe cerebral palsy by age 2, and other maternal and neonatal complications.

RESULTS

- Exposure to magnesium sulfate in utero was not associated with a reduction of the primary composite outcome of intrauterine death, death prior to a year of life, or moderate to moderate/severe cerebral palsy. (See Table 10.1.) One or more of the events that comprise the primary outcome occurred in 11.3% of pregnancies in the magnesium arm and 11.7% of pregnancies in the placebo arm (relative risk [RR] 0.97, 95% confidence interval [CI] 0.77–1.23).
- Among survivors, there was a lower risk of moderate/severe cerebral palsy following in utero magnesium exposure compared to placebo (1.9% vs. 3.5%, RR 0.55, 95% CI 0.32–0.95, $p = 0.03$).
- Stillbirth or death within the first year of life was not significantly different between the two arms of the trial (9.5% vs. 8.5%, RR 1.12, 95% 0.85–1.47).
- In stratified analyses, benefits of magnesium sulfate in terms of reducing moderate/cerebral palsy were demonstrated only in those randomized <28 weeks gestation:
  - <28 weeks: 2.7% vs. 6.0%, RR 0.45, 95% CI 0.23–0.87
  - ≥28 weeks: 1.3% vs. 1.3%, RR 1.00, 95% CI 0.38–2.65

Table 10.1. Outcomes

Outcome	Magnesium Sulfate ($n = 1041$)	Placebo ($n = 1095$)	Relative Risk (95% Confidence Interval)	p-value
All participants				
Moderate or severe cerebral palsy or death	118/1041 (11.3%)	128/1095 (11.7%)	0.97 (0.77–1.23)	0.80
Moderate or severe cerebral palsy alone	20/1041 (1.9%)	38/1095 (3.5%)	0.55 (0.32–0.95)	0.03
Death alone	99/1041 (9.5%)	93/1095 (8.5%)	1.12 (0.85–1.47)	0.41

Criticisms and Limitations: Based on the exclusion criteria, the majority of enrolled patients had preterm premature rupture of membranes (~86%) and the use of tocolysis after randomized was not allowed. This may limit the generalizability of these findings. Furthermore, the sample size may have been too small to detect a difference in outcomes, as they overestimated the expected rate of moderate or severe cerebral palsy.

Other Relevant Studies and Information:

- The hypothesis that magnesium sulfate may have neuroprotective effects initially stemmed from observational studies in which a lower rate of neurologic injury was noted among infants exposed to magnesium sulfate in utero.[2]
- Three randomized trials predating BEAM, all of which included a smaller number of participants and with slightly different magnesium protocols, were similarly unable to demonstrate a reduction in a primary composite outcome of death or cerebral palsy/neurologic injury.[3-5]
- A subsequent individual patient-level data meta-analysis was published in 2017 summarizing the results of these 4 four randomized controlled trials in which magnesium sulfate was used antenatally with neuroprotective intent and did demonstrate a reduction in the composite of death or cerebral palsy (RR 0.86, 95% CI 0.75–0.99, n = 4,488 infants, 4 trials).[6] The risk of cerebral palsy among surviving infants, when considered as an outcome alone, was also significantly reduced in this meta-analysis (RR 0.68, 95% CI 0.53–0.87, n = 3988 infants, 4 trials). The number needed to treat to prevent 1 death or infant affected by cerebral palsy was 1 in 41. The authors also note there was little variation in the effect of magnesium sulfate when evaluated by gestational age administered, underlying etiology of the preterm birth, total dose administered, or dosing regimen utilized (e.g., bolus alone or with maintenance).
- The American College of Obstetricians and Gynecologists and the Society for Maternal-Fetal Medicine guidelines suggest that it is reasonable for physicians to consider magnesium sulfate for fetal neuroprotection during pregnancies at risk for preterm birth given the evidence of benefit among surviving infants. Guidelines do not dictate specific dosing regimens or length of treatment, although it is reasonable to offer this intervention up to 32 weeks of gestation in line with BEAM inclusion criteria.

Summary and Implications: The BEAM trial was the largest randomized controlled trial designed specifically to evaluate the neuroprotective impact of antenatal magnesium sulfate administered to women at risk of preterm birth. The trial did not demonstrate a benefit of magnesium sulfate for preventing a composite of adverse outcomes, including stillbirth, but did demonstrate a reduced risk of cerebral palsy among surviving infants by an estimated 45%. Based on these results and other studies, magnesium sulfate should be considered for fetal neuroprotection during pregnancies at risk for preterm birth less than 32 weeks.

CLINICAL CASE: ROLE OF MAGNESIUM FOR FETAL NEUROPROTECTION

Case History

A 31-year-old G2P1 at 28 weeks and 2 days presents to the labor and delivery floor with leakage of clear fluid. Her initial speculum exam confirms spontaneous rupture of membranes and cervical dilation of 5cm. The fetal testing is reassuring on nonstress test. Tocometry shows contractions every 5 to 7 minutes, and the patient appears mildly uncomfortable. How should the patient be counseled on possible fetal outcomes? What interventions would you recommend given this initial presentation?

Suggested Answer

For patients presenting with preterm premature rupture of membranes, regular contractions, and cervical dilation, there is concern for imminent preterm delivery. In addition to standard recommendations, including steroids for fetal lung maturity, the patient should be counseled on the risk of neonatal complications associated with prematurity. Additionally, she should be counseled on the anticipated benefit of magnesium given her gestational age would meet the inclusion criteria utilized in the BEAM trial (<32 weeks). We would recommend proceeding with a 6g bolus of magnesium followed by a 2g maintenance infusion as utilized in BEAM. If the patient does not progress in labor, it would be reasonable to discontinue the magnesium after a period of observation.

References

1. Rouse DJ, Hirtz DG, Thom E, et al. A randomized, controlled trial of magnesium sulfate for the prevention of cerebral palsy. *N Engl J Med.* 2008;359(9):895–905. doi:10.1056/NEJMoa0801187

2. Caddell JL, Graziani LJ, Wiswell TE, Hsieh HC, Mansmann HC Jr. The possible role of magnesium in protection of premature infants from neurological syndromes

and visual impairments and a review of survival of magnesium-exposed premature infants. *Magnes Res.* 1999;12(3):201–216.

3. Mittendorf R, Dambrosia J, Pryde PG, Lee KS, Gianopoulos JG, Besinger RE, et al. Association between the use of antenatal magnesium sulfate in preterm labor and adverse health outcomes in infants. *Am J Obstet Gynecol.* 2002;186(6):1111–1118.

4. Crowther CA, Hiller JE, Doyle LW, Haslnbam RR. Effect of magnesium sulfate given for neuroprotection before preterm birth: a randomized controlled trial. Australian Collaborative Trial of Magnesium Sulfate (ACTOMgSO4) Collaborative Group. *JAMA.* 2003;290:2669–2676.

5. Marret S, Marpeau L, Follet-Bouhamed C, Cambonie G, Astruc D, Delaporte B, et al. Effect of magnesium sulphate on mortality and neurologic morbidity of the very-preterm newborn (of less than 33 weeks) with two-year neurological out-come: results of the prospective PREMAG trial. Le groupe PREMAG [French]. *Gynecol Obstet Fertil.* 2008;36:278–288.

6. Crowther CA, Middleton PF, Voysey M, Askie L, Duley L, Pryde PG, Marret S, Doyle LM, for the AMICABLE Group. Assessing the neuroprotective benefits for babies of antenatal magnesium sulfate: an individual participant data meta-analysis. *PLoS Med.* 2017;14(10):e1002398.

7. Society for Maternal-Fetal Medicine. Magnesium sulfate before anticipated pre-term birth for neuroprotection. Committee Opinion no. 455. *Obstet Gynecol.* 2010;115:669–671.

11

Pelvic Scoring for Elective Induction

The Bishop Score

C. SOLA AJEWOLE AND JODI F. ABBOTT

"Therefore, it would seem of benefit to develop some standardized, easily determined, and easily recorded plan for the selection of those patients most suitable for induction, hopefully resulting in acceptable outcomes for all."

—E BISHOP[1]

Research Question: Is there a standard method to select patients suitable for elective induction?

Funding: None

Year Study Began: 1950

Year Study Published: 1964

Location: Pennsylvania Hospital, Philadelphia, Pennsylvania

Who Was Studied: Multiparous women at 36 weeks or greater, vertex presentation, and an uncomplicated obstetric history.

Who Was Excluded: None listed

How Many Patients: 500

Study Overview: This study was a prospective observational study intended to evaluate the average duration of pregnancy from time of vaginal examination (assessing dilation, effacement, station, consistency, and position) to spontaneous onset of labor.

Follow-Up: 35 days

Endpoints: Primary outcome was average duration of pregnancy from time of examination to the spontaneous onset of labor

---

RESULTS

- The findings illustrated that in a population of 500 uncomplicated patients, a higher pelvic score correlated with a shorter interval to spontaneous labor. See Figure 9.1.
- The authors indicated that, in their experience, induction was most successful in patients with a Bishop score greater than 9, claiming no failures of induction and an average duration of 4 hours or less of labor. Of note, data was not presented in the paper to support this statement.

Criticisms and Limitations: The observational study was written in 1964; standards for presentation of evidence and data differed. The paper does present what could be considered pilot, observational data that supports the development of the Bishop score, although more current methods of scale development might rely on factor analysis or tests for internal and external validity that are not applied here.

It is important to note that the authors conclude that the pelvic score can be used to determine the optimal time for induction, but that finding is not based on data presented in this paper, as the presented data only demonstrates time to spontaneous labor.

The validity of the scale to other populations is also not clear, as the included patients met a fairly narrow set of inclusion criteria (multiparous, full-term, vertex, and uncomplicated).

Other Relevant Studies and Information:

- Several studies have been published to validate the use of the score in clinical practice. Bishop and colleagues published results comparing methods of induction among 1000 multiparous women who were selected using the score presented.[2] This study found that delaying induction would result in more "favorable" pelvic exams with shorter labors and identified a "favorable" exam as 3cm dilated, 70% effaced, and at least 1 station.

- A later iteration of the Bishop score was simplified to only 3 components (dilation, effacement, and station) and found to have the same predictive value for spontaneous vaginal delivery as the full Bishop score (Table 11.1).[3] This study included a large number of nulliparous patients, making it more generalizable.

Table 11.1. ORIGINAL BISHOP SCORE

Pelvic Score Points	0	1	2	3
Dilation (cm)	0	1–2	3–4	5–6
Effacement (%)	0–30	40–50	60–70	80
Station	−3	−2	−1, 0	+1, +2
Consistency	Firm	Medium	Soft	-
Position	Posterior	Middle	Anterior	-

This table demonstrates the information that was ascertained from vaginal examination as well as the point(s) assigned for each finding. At the time of this publication, a score of 9 or greater meant induction could be successfully and safely performed.

- Additional studies have found that this score predicted the success of a vaginal deliveries in women with nonelective indications for inductions both at term and preterm, as well as determining that an unfavorable cervix (defined as a Bishops score less than or equal to 5 had an increased need for oxytocin augmentation and increased rates of cesarean delivery.[3,4]
- Currently, the American College of Obstetricians and Gynecologists advocates for utilizing a full Bishop score when assessing the cervix as a tool for determining which patients are candidates for cervical ripening including those attempting a vaginal birth after cesarean (VBAC).[5,6]

Summary and Implications: In this study, the authors provided validation for a cervical scoring system that identified the cervical characteristics that predict onset of labor. The Bishop score has been subsequently utilized as a tool for assessing readiness for labor induction. This score has since been validated as a tool to guide induction method through randomized controlled trials; later studies, too, have also confirmed its utility in nulliparous patients.

CLINICAL CASE

Case History

A 26-year-old G2P1 presents at 39 weeks by last menstrual period consistent with an ultrasound completed at 8 weeks. This pregnancy is complicated by a recent diagnosis of gestational hypertension. In light of her diagnosis, it is recommended she have an induction of labor. A cervical exam is performed, and she is found to be 1cm/30%/–3/medium/posterior, correlating to a pelvic (Bishop) score of 2.

Based on the results of Bishop's study of pelvic scoring, what intervention would you recommend to initiate her induction?

Suggested Answer

The Bishop score has proven to be a useful tool for predicting successful vaginal delivery in patients requiring induction. Cervical ripening is indicated in this patient, as currently her probability of successful labor is low.

References

1. Bishop EH. Pelvic Scoring for Elective Induction. *Obstet Gynecol.* 1964;24(2):266–268. PMID:14199536.
2. Bishop EH. Elective Induction of Labor. *Obstet Gynecol.* 1955;5(4):519–527. PMID:14370696.
3. Laughon SK, Zhang J, Troendle J, Sun L, Reddy UM. Using a simplified bishop core to predict vaginal delivery. *Obstet Gynecol.* 2011;117(4):805–811. https://doi.org/10.1097/AOG.0b013e3182114ad2
4. Raghuraman N, Stout MJ, Young OM, Tuuli MG, López JD, MacOnes GA, Cahill AG. Utility of the simplified bishop score in spontaneous labor. *Am J Perinatol.* 2016;33(12):1176–1181. https://doi.org/10.1055/s-0036-1585413
5. Shields LE, Goffman D, Caughey AB. ACOG practice bulletin: clinical management guidelines for obstetrician-gynecologists. *Obstet Gynecol.* 2017;130(4):e168–e186. https://doi.org/10.1097/AOG.0000000000002351
6. Metz TD, Stoddard GJ, Henry E, Jackson M, Holmgren C, Esplin S. Simple, validated vaginal birth after cesarean delivery prediction model for use at the time of admission. *Obstet Gynecol.* 2013;122(3):571–578. https://doi.org/10.1097/AOG.0b013e31829f8ced

12

Management of Post-Term Pregnancy

The Post-Term Pregnancy Trial

ASHLEY E. BENSON AND BRETT D. EINERSON

"Inducing labor in women with post-term pregnancies results in a decrease in the rate of cesarean section as compared with serial antenatal monitoring and no difference in the incidence of perinatal mortality and neonatal morbidity."

—ME Hannah[1]

Research Question: Should patients with post-term pregnancies at 41 weeks' gestation or greater be managed with induction of labor or serial antenatal monitoring?

Funding: Medical Research Council of Canada.

Year Study Began: 1985

Year Study Published: 1992

Study Location: 22 hospitals in Canada

Who Was Studied: Pregnant women with a single, live fetus who had reached 41+ weeks' gestation by standardized dating criteria available at the time.

Who Was Excluded: Patients with comorbid diabetes, preeclampsia, substance abuse (alcohol or drugs), intrauterine growth restriction, or prelabor rupture of membranes were excluded. Additional exclusion criteria were gestational age ≥44 weeks, cervical dilation ≥3cm, need for urgent delivery, prior cesarean, contraindication to vaginal delivery, noncephalic presentation, and anomalous fetuses.

How Many Patients: 3,407

Study Overview: This was a randomized controlled trial. See Figure 12.1

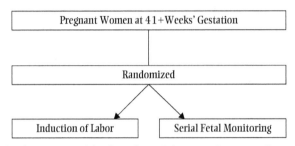

Figure 12.1. Study overview: The Canadian Multicenter Post-term Pregnancy Trial

Study Intervention: Patients randomized to the induction group were induced within 4 days. If the cervix was <3cm or <50% effaced and there was normal fetal heart rate, Prostaglandin E2 gel was given. After insertion, fetal monitoring was performed for a minimum of 1 hour. Over 6-hour intervals, a maximum of 3 doses of E2 gel could be given. If gel was not used or it did not induce labor, oxytocin +/– amniotomy was performed. Oxytocin was started 12 hours after last insertion of gel.

Women randomized to the monitoring group recorded kick counts and underwent fetal non-stress test (NST) 3 times per week with amniotic fluid volume (AFV) measurement 2 to 3 times per week. Women with fewer than 6 kicks in 2 hours were to contact their physician and undergo NST within 12 hours. In the setting of nonreactive NST or low AFV (pocket <3cm), obstetrical complications, or gestational age >44 weeks, patients were immediately delivered either via induction (with amniotomy or oxytocin) or cesarean section.

Continuous fetal monitoring was performed during labor for both groups. Mode of delivery was determined by the attending physician. Cord-blood gases, cord-blood hematocrit, and Apgar scores were obtained. The physicians managing the infants were aware of the labor management method.

Follow-Up: Until time of hospital discharge

Endpoints: Primary outcomes: Perinatal mortality (stillbirth or neonatal death before discharge) and neonatal morbidity index score (derived from expert consensus and comprised several factors including Apgar scores, birth weight, need for resuscitation, base deficit, and presence of meconium, as well as other factors. Secondary outcomes: A number of individual neonatal and maternal outcomes included in the indices noted previously.

RESULTS

- 24.5% of women had a cesarean section in the serial monitoring group versus 21.2% in the induction group with an odds ratio of 1.22 (95% confidence interval 1.02–1.45) (Table 12.1).
- 8.3% of women underwent cesarean section due to fetal distress in the serial monitoring group versus 5.7% in the induction group.
- There were no differences in perinatal mortality or neonatal morbidity between study groups (Table 12.1).
- There were 2 stillbirths in the serial monitoring group, although the study was underpowered to evaluate this outcome.

Table 12.1. SUMMARY OF KEY FINDINGS

Outcome	Serial Monitoring Group	Induction Group	*p*-value
Cesarean Delivery (CD)	24.5%	21.2%	0.03
CD Due to Fetal Distress	8.3%	5.7%	0.003
Neonatal Morbidity	2.1%	2.3%	0.643

Abbreviation: CD, Cesarean Delivery.

Criticisms and Limitations: The study had suboptimal protocol adherence, with only 66% of the patients randomized to induction undergoing induction, effectively being managed instead by serial monitoring. The providers were also unblinded to randomized and thus may have been more likely to perform cesarean delivery for fetal distress in the monitoring group.

Other Relevant Studies and Information:

- A cost-minimization analysis of the same cohort demonstrated induction of labor to manage post-term pregnancy not only results in more favorable outcomes, compared to serial monitoring, but does so at decreased cost.[2]

- A recent meta-analysis demonstrated that post-term induction of labor is associated with fewer perinatal deaths, fewer newborn intensive care unit admissions, and fewer cesarean sections.[3]

- Since the publication of this study, Canada has seen a decrease in stillbirth rates, attributed in part to a reduced proportion of births at 42 or more weeks.[4]

- A recent randomized controlled trial investigated outcomes for IOL at 39 weeks versus expectant management in low-risk nulliparous women without indication for induction (ARRIVE Trial). The study found no significant difference in the primary outcome of perinatal outcomes; however, there was lower rate of primary cesarean deliveries and in hypertensive disorders of pregnancy. These data further support the conclusion that IOL at term may decrease the risk of cesarean.[5]

- The American College of Obstetricians and Gynecologists recommends induction of labor between 42 $0/7$ and 42 $6/7$ (Level A recommendation) due to increased perinatal mortality and morbidity; induction between 41 $0/7$ and 41 $6/7$ can be considered (Level B recommendation).[6]

Summary and Implications: In pregnancies of 41+ weeks' gestation, induction of labor results in fewer cesarean sections overall, specifically fewer cesarean sections for fetal distress compared with serial antenatal testing. These results apply to singleton pregnancies without maternal or fetal comorbidities. Neonatal morbidity and mortality were not significantly different. This study, the findings of which have subsequently been confirmed in other studies, is the foundation for commonly employed guidelines recommending induction of labor at 41+ weeks' gestation.

CLINICAL CASE: INDUCTION OF LABOR FOR POST-TERM PREGNANCIES

Case History

A 34-year-old G2P1001 presents to you at 40 weeks' gestation for routine prenatal care. You suggest induction of labor if she has not had spontaneous labor by 41 weeks. The patient is hesitant, expressing that she would prefer the process to be as natural as possible. Based on the results of the induction of labor compared with serial antenatal monitoring in post-term pregnancy trial, how would you counsel her?

Suggested Answer

The Post-Term trial demonstrated that induction of labor in pregnancies of 41 or greater weeks' gestation results in fewer cesarean sections, especially those done for fetal distress. There was no significant difference in neonatal outcome between the two groups.

The patient in this vignette should be recommended to undergo induction of labor if she has not labored by 41 weeks. If she declines, she should continue to be monitored with weekly NSTs and AFI. After appropriate counseling, she should be able to describe an increased risk of fetal distress in labor and cesarean section with ongoing expectant management beyond 41 weeks.

References

1. Hannah ME, Hannah WJ, Hellmann J, Hewson S, Milner R, Willan A. Induction of labor as compared with serial antenatal monitoring in post-term pregnancy: a randomized controlled trial. The Canadian Multicenter Post-Term Pregnancy Trial Group. *N Engl J Med.* 1992;326(24):1587–1592.
2. Goeree R, Hannah M, Hewson S. Cost-effectiveness of induction of labour versus serial antenatal monitoring in the Canadian Multicentre Postterm Pregnancy Trial. *CMAJ.* 1995;152(9):1445–1450.
3. Middleton P, Shepherd E, Crowther CA. Induction of labour for improving birth outcomes for women at or beyond term. *Cochrane Database Syst Rev.* 2018;5:Cd004945.
4. Sue AQAK, Hannah ME, Cohen MM, Foster GA, Liston, RM. Effect of labour induction on rates of stillbirth and cesarean section in post-term pregnancies. *CMAJ.* 1999;160(8):1145–1149.
5. Grobman WA, Rice MM, Reddy UM, Tita AT, Silver RM, Mallett G, et al. Labor induction versus expectant management in low-risk nulliparous women. Eunice Kennedy Shriver National Institute of Child Health and Human Development Maternal–Fetal Medicine Units Network. *N Engl J Med.* 2018;379:513–523.
6. American College of Obstetricians and Gynecologists. Practice bulletin no. 146: management of late-term and postterm pregnancies. *Obstet Gynecol.* 2014; 124(2 Pt 1): 390–396. doi:10.1097/01.AOG.0000452744.06088.48

13

Planned Cesarean Section Versus Planned Vaginal Birth for Breech Presentation at Term

The Term Breech Trial

SAMANTHA MORRISON AND HUGH EHRENBERG

"Planned cesarean section is better than planned vaginal birth for the term fetus in the breech presentation; serious maternal complications are similar between the groups."

—ME HANNAH ET AL.[1]

Research Question: Is planned cesarean section better than planned vaginal birth at term for singleton non-anomalous fetuses with breech presentation at term?

Funding: The Canadian Institutes of Health Research. Data coordinating center support from the Centre for Research in Women's Health, Sunnybrook and Women's College Health Sciences Centre and the University of Toronto

Year Study Began: 1997

Year Study Published: 2000

Study Location: 121 centers in 26 countries

Who Was Studied: Women with a singleton live fetus in a frank or complete breech presentation at term (≥37 weeks)

Who Was Excluded: Estimated fetal weight (EFW) >4000g or fetopelvic disproportion, hyperextension of the fetal head, known lethal fetal congenital anomaly, contraindication to either labor or vaginal delivery

How Many Patients: 2,088

Study Overview: This was a randomized controlled trial. See Figure 13.1

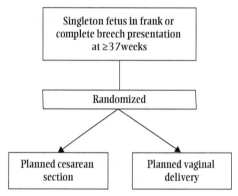

Figure 13.1 Study overview: The Term Breech Trial

Study Intervention: Patients were assigned to either the planned cesarean group (CS) or the planned vaginal birth group (VD). In the planned CS group, delivery was arranged at 38 or more weeks' gestation, or earlier if the patient presented in labor. Fetal position was reassessed immediately prior to surgery and, if cephalic, vaginal birth was planned. Greater than 90% of this group was expected to deliver by CS. In the planned VD group, pregnancy was managed with expectant management until spontaneous labor, unless induction or immediate CS was medically indicated. Only complete or frank breech presentation was managed in this fashion. An experienced clinician, defined by the local department chair, was to be present at every delivery. CS was undertaken for fetal heart rate abnormalities or prolonged labor. The fetal head was delivered via forceps or the Mauriceau-Smellie-Veit maneuver. Breech extraction was prohibited. Greater than 50% of these patients were expected to deliver vaginally.

Follow-Up: 6 weeks post-partum

Endpoints: Primary outcomes included perinatal or neonatal mortality at less than 28 days of age (excluding lethal congenital anomalies) or serious neonatal morbidity. Secondary outcomes included maternal mortality or serious maternal morbidity within the first 6 weeks post-partum.

RESULTS

- 90.4% of women randomized to the planned CS group delivered by CS, and 56.7% of women randomized to the VD group delivered vaginally. Reasons for unscheduled CS in the VD group included labor dystocia, fetal heart rate tracing abnormalities, cord prolapse, and footling breech.
- There was a significantly lower risk of the combined outcome of perinatal/ neonatal mortality or serious neonatal morbidity in the planned CS group (1.6%) than in the planned VD group (5.0%, see Table 13.1).
- There were no significant differences between the two groups in terms of maternal mortality or serious maternal morbidity.
- The reduction in risk attributable to planned CS was greatest among centers in industrialized nations with low overall perinatal mortality rates (0.4 vs. 5.7%). There were no significant interactions between treatment group and maternal age, parity, type of breech presentation, gestational age, presence of labor, EFW, ruptured membranes, or standard of care provided by the center.

Table 13.1. Perinatal or Neonatal Mortality at <28 Days of Age and Serious Neonatal Morbidity for the Planned CS Cesarean Group Versus the Planned VD

Perinatal/ Neonatal Outcome	CS	VD	Relative Risk (95% CI)	p-value
Perinatal/neonatal mortality or serious neonatal morbidity	17/1039 (1.6%)	52/1039 (5.0%)	0.33 (0.19–0.56)	<0.0001
Perinatal/neonatal mortality	3/1039 (0.3%)	13/1039 (1.3%)	0.23 (0.07–0.81)	0.01
Serious neonatal morbidity	14/1036 (1.4%)	39/1026 (3.8%)	0.36 (0.19–0.65)	0.0003
Maternal mortality or serious morbidity	41/1041 (3.9%)	33/1042 (3.2%)	1.24 (0.79–1.95)	0.35

Abbreviations: CS, cesarean group; VD, vaginal delivery group; CI, confidence interval.

- A policy of planned CS for breech infants at term avoids death or serious morbidity in 1 neonate for every additional 14 CS performed.
- Following the second interim analysis, recruitment was ended due to the significantly lower rate of perinatal mortality in patients randomized to planned cesarean section.

Criticisms and Limitations:

- Many of the centers involved in this trial were in North America where the term vaginal breech delivery rate was only 13%. To qualify for this trial, these centers had to increase their breech vaginal delivery rate significantly. This increase would constitute a significant bias due to a lack of experienced and skilled practitioners available to undertake vaginal breech deliveries.[2] Furthermore, many of the vaginal stillbirths were due to fetal heart rate abnormalities and inability to deliver by CS. This highlights variation in the standard of care between participating centers.
- This study did not address the long-term risks of CS on maternal health and the risks in subsequent pregnancies.

Other Relevant Studies and Information:

- Within a few months of publication of the Term Birth Trial, obstetric practice worldwide was transformed. In 2001, the American College of Obstetricians and Gynecologists' (ACOG) stated planned vaginal delivery of a term singleton breech was no longer appropriate.[3] A survey of term breech trial collaborators, from 80 centers in 23 countries, reported a 92.5% changed rate in clinical practice to planned cesarean birth for all term breech babies.[4]
- In August 2018 ACOG updated its recommendations to emphasize that all patients with a breech presentation should be offered external cephalic version if appropriate and that planned vaginal delivery of a term singleton breech fetus may be reasonable under specific circumstances, taking into account the patient's wishes and the experience of the health care provider.[5]

Summary and Implications: The Term Breech Trial showed that, for singleton fetuses in the breech presentation at term, a policy of planned cesarean section is superior to attempting vaginal delivery, with the benefits greatest in countries with lower perinatal mortality rates. A policy of planned cesarean section is not associated with a higher risk of serious maternal complications in the first 6 weeks post-partum.

CLINICAL CASE: DELIVERY OF THE BREECH FETUS AT TERM

Case History

A 33-year-old G3P2002 at 37 weeks gestation presents for induction of labor secondary to gestational hypertension. She has no other medical problems. Her obstetric history is significant for 2 full-term, uncomplicated spontaneous vaginal deliveries. Ultrasound confirms a singleton fetus in frank breech presentation with an EFW of 3250g. Elective external cephalic version is unsuccessful. She would like to know what mode of delivery is safest for her and her baby. Based on the results of the this trial, how should this patient be counseled?

Suggested Answer

The Term Breech Trial was a large multicenter randomized controlled trial that concluded that a planned cesarean delivery compared to breech vaginal birth reduces perinatal/neonatal mortality and serious neonatal morbidity by 68% (1.6% vs. 5%, relative risk 0.33), without significantly increasing the risk of serious maternal morbidity and mortality. Based on these findings, the "safest" mode of delivery is planned cesarean section. She should be offered the option of an external cephalic version and can be offered a breech vaginal delivery if she is deemed an appropriate candidate and an experienced provider is present for delivery.

References

1. Hannah ME, Hannah WJ, Hewson SA, Hodnett ED, Saigal S, Willan AR. Planned caesarean section versus planned vaginal birth for breech presentation at term: a randomised multicentre trial. Term Breech Trial Collaborative Group. *Lancet.* 2000;356(9239):1375–1383. doi:10.1016/s0140-6736(00)02840-3
2. Kotaska A. Inappropriate use of randomised trials to evaluate complex phenomena: case study of vaginal breech delivery. *BMJ.* 2004;329(7473):1039–1042.
3. American College of Obstetricians and Gynecologists. *Mode of term singelton breech delivery.* American College of Obstetricians and Gynecologists Committee Opinion No 265. 2001. Washington, DC.
4. Hogle KL, Kilburn L, Hewson S, Gafni A, Wall R, Hannah, ME. Impact of the international term breech trial on clinical practice and concerns: a survey of centre collaborators. *J Obstet Gynaecol Can.* 2003;25(1):14–16.
5. American College of Obstetricians and Gynecologists. *Mode of term singleton breech delivery.* American College of Obstetricians and Gynecologists Committee Opinion No 745. 2018. Washington, DC.

14

Induction of Labor Versus Expectant Management for Prelabor Rupture of Membranes

The TERMPROM Study

ADINA KERN-GOLDBERGER AND DENA GOFFMAN

"Induction of labor with intravenous oxytocin, induction of labor with vaginal prostaglandin E_2 gel, and expectant management are all reasonable options for women and their babies if membranes rupture before the start of labor at term."

—THE TERMPROM STUDY GROUP[1]

Research Question: Should prelabor rupture of membranes at term be managed with induction of labor or expectantly?

Funding: Medical Research Council of Canada

Year Study Began: 1992

Year Study Published: 1996

Study Location: 72 hospitals in Canada, the United Kingdom, Australia, Israel, Sweden, and Denmark

Who Was Studied: Pregnant women with prelabor rupture of membranes at ≥37 weeks gestation

Who Was Excluded: Patients in active labor, patients with history of prior failed induction of labor, patients with contraindication to labor induction, and patients with contraindication to expectant management (meconium-stained amniotic fluid, chorioamnionitis)

How Many Patients: 5,042

Study Overview: This was a randomized controlled trial. See Figure 14.1

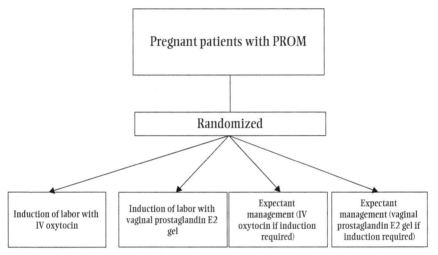

Figure 14.1. Study overview: The TERMPROM Study

Study Intervention: All patients had a fetal non-stress test and group B streptococci (GBS) swab prior to enrollment. During the time period of this study, GBS was not routinely swabbed during antenatal care. Patients in the oxytocin induction group received intravenous (IV) oxytocin through an infusion titrated according to local hospital practice. Patients in the prostaglandin E_2 gel induction received 1mg or 2mg of prostaglandin E_2 gel inserted in the posterior vaginal fornix, which was repeated 6 hours later if labor had not yet started and was followed by an oxytocin infusion 4 or more hours later if labor still had not commenced.

Patients in the expectant management group were either admitted to the hospital or managed as outpatients. The patients monitored their temperature twice daily and reported any fevers or changes in the color and odor of the amniotic fluid. If complications developed or labor did not start after 4 days, labor was induced with either oxytocin or prostaglandin E_2 gel in the same way as it was induced for the induction groups.

Endpoints: Primary outcome: Neonatal infection (definite or probable based on clinical signs of infection and correlating laboratory or microbiological results). Secondary outcomes: Cesarean section; patient's subjective evaluation of the care they received; and other measures of maternal, fetal, and neonatal health including perinatal mortality, chorioamnionitis, postpartum maternal fever, neonatal antibiotics, and neonatal intensive care admission

---

RESULTS

- The majority of patients in the induction groups were induced (89.0% in the oxytocin induction group and 89.7% in the prostaglandin induction group); labor began spontaneously in the majority of patients in the expectant management groups (77.0% in the oxytocin expectant management group and 78.5% in the prostaglandin expectant-management group).
- There was no difference in the rate of neonatal infection across all four groups (2.0% in the oxytocin induction group, 3.0% in the prostaglandin E_2 gel group, 2.8% in the expectant management [oxytocin] group, and 2.7% in the expectant management [prostaglandin] group). (See Table 14.1.)

Table 14.1. SUMMARY OF TERMPROM's KEY FINDINGS

Induction with Oxytocin vs. Expectant Management

Outcome	Induction with Oxytocin n (%)	Expectant Management (Oxytocin) n %	Odds Ratio (95% Confidence Interval)
Neonatal infection	25 (2.0)	36 (2.8)	0.7 (0.4–1.2)
Cesarean section	127 (10.1)	123 (9.7)	1.0 (0.8–1.4)

Induction with Oxytocin vs. Induction with Prostaglandin

Outcome	Induction with Oxytocin n (%)	Induction with Prostaglandin n (%)	Odds Ratio (95% Confidence Interval)
Neonatal infection	25 (2.0)	38 (3.0)	1.5 (0.9–2.6)
Cesarean section	127 (10.1)	121 (9.6)	1.0 (0.7–1.2)

- There was also no difference in the rate of cesarean section across all 4 groups (10.1% in the oxytocin induction group, 9.6% in the prostaglandin E_2 gel group, 9.7% in the expectant management [oxytocin] group, and 10.9% in the expectant management [prostaglandin] group).
- The incidence of chorioamnionitis was 4.0% in the oxytocin induction group compared to 8.6% in the expectant management (oxytocin) group ($p < 0.01$); postpartum fever occurred in 1.9% of patients induced with oxytocin compared to expectant management (oxytocin) at 3.6% ($p < 0.01$).
- Patients in the oxytocin induction group had fewer digital vaginal examinations, earlier onset of active labor, shorter labor courses, shorter interval between membrane rupture and delivery, and less time in the hospital prior to delivery than patients in the prostaglandin E_2 gel induction and expectant management (oxytocin) groups.
- More women in the induction groups said that if they were in the same position again, they would participate in the study and were less likely to say they liked "nothing" about their treatment compared to the expectant management group (oxytocin).

Criticisms and Limitations: The trial recommended (but did not require) intrapartum antibiotic treatment of patients with positive GBS swabs, which is now considered standard of clinical care, and only a minority of GBS positive patients actually received antibiotics in the study. Now that all patients with GBS receive routine intrapartum prophylaxis, these data may no longer apply.

In addition, the randomization to method of induction or to expectant management was made independent of initial cervical exam (or without one in >60% of participants); however, in clinical practice, the initial cervical exam may play an important role in the decision for induction versus expectant management and in method of induction, as well as in the potential efficacy of the management.

It is also difficult to draw conclusions about neonatal treatments such as antibiotic administration and neonatal intensive care admission as these may have been influenced by greater caregiver concern for neonates born to women whose membranes were ruptured for longer periods.

The results of this study differ from other randomized controlled trials that have indicated a lower risk of neonatal infection when labor is induced shortly after membrane rupture as well as an association between induction and risk of cesarean section.[2-4]

Other Relevant Studies and Information:

- Several further analyses of the TERMPROM trial have demonstrated that clinical chorioamnionitis and positive maternal GBS swab are the best predictors of neonatal infection; induction of labor with IV oxytocin may be preferable for women who are GBS positive as compared to induction with prostaglandin or expectant management; and expectant management at home, rather than a hospital, may increase the risk of adverse outcomes.[5,6]
- No other large randomized trials of this scale have been conducted evaluating induction compared to expectant management and comparing oxytocin to prostaglandin for induction of labor in the setting of prelabor rupture of membranes (PROM). Several meta-analyses have demonstrated supportive findings including evidence suggesting that induction lowers the risk of maternal infectious morbidity compared to expectant management without an increase in the rate of cesarean section and comparable rates of neonatal complications among women with PROM induced with oxytocin compared to prostaglandin.[7,8]
- Newer research has focused on the role of mechanical cervical ripening in the setting of PROM, with multiple randomized controlled trials demonstrating no decrease in time to delivery with concurrent intracervical Foley catheter and oxytocin compared to oxytocin alone, with a possible increase in the incidence of chorioamnionitis.[9,10]
- For women at term with PROM, the American College of Obstetricians and Gynecologists recommends delivery (induction or cesarean section as clinically appropriate) and GBS prophylaxis as indicated.[11]

Summary and Implications: In patients with PROM at term, induction of labor with intravenous oxytocin, vaginal prostaglandin E_2 gel, or expectant management are all reasonable options with similar rates of neonatal infection and cesarean section. However, induction of labor with IV oxytocin is associated with a lower risk of maternal infection than expectant management and women have more positive experiences intrapartum with induction after rupture of membranes versus expectant management.

CLINICAL CASE: INDUCTION OF LABOR VERSUS EXPECTANT MANAGEMENT IN PROM

Case History

A 34-year old G1P0 at 40 weeks presents to obstetric triage complaining of ruptured membranes 6 hours prior. She is comfortable and not contracting. Pelvic exam confirms rupture of membranes by positive nitrazine swab and fluid pooling as well a long, closed cervix. Her GBS swab is positive and fetal non-stress test is reactive.

Based on the results of TERMPROM, how should this patient be treated?

Suggested Answer

TERMPROM demonstrated that induction with oxytocin, induction with vaginal prostaglandin, and expectant management are all acceptable options for management of PROM at term in regards to risk for neonatal infection and cesarean section. Although there is no difference in neonatal infection, the risk for chorioamnionitis and postpartum maternal fever is higher with expectant management as compared to induction with oxytocin. Therefore, oxytocin induction may be the better option for this patient.

TERMPROM did not, however, account for GBS status or starting cervical exam. Maternal positive GBS swab has subsequently been demonstrated to predict neonatal infection, and research has suggested that induction with oxytocin may be better than expectant management or induction with vaginal prostaglandin for these patients, further encouraging the use of oxytocin for induction in this case.

References

1. Hannah ME, Ohlsson A, Farine D, et al. Induction of labor compared with expectant management for prelabor rupture of the membranes at term. TERMPROM Study Group. *N Engl J Med.* 1996;334(16):1005–1010. doi:10.1056/NEJM199604183341601
2. Duff P, Huff RW, Gibbs, RS. Management of premature rupture of membranes and unfavorable cervix in term pregnancy. *Obstet Gynecol.* 1984;63(5):697–702.
3. Hauth JC, Cunningham FG, Whalley, PJ. Early labor initiation with oral PGE2 after premature rupture of the membranes at term. *Obstet Gynecol.* 1977;49(5):523–526.
4. Wagner MV, et al. A comparison of early and delayed induction of labor with spontaneous rupture of membranes at term. *Obstet Gynecol.* 1989;74(1):93–97.

5. Hannah ME, et al. Maternal colonization with group B Streptococcus and prelabor rupture of membranes at term: the role of induction of labor. TermPROM Study Group. *Am J Obstet Gynecol.* 1997;177(4):780–785.

6. Hannah ME, et al. Prelabor rupture of the membranes at term: expectant management at home or in hospital? The TermPROM Study Group. *Obstet Gynecol.* 2000;96(4):533–538.

7. Middleton P, et al. Planned early birth versus expectant management (waiting) for prelabour rupture of membranes at term (37 weeks or more). *Cochrane Database Syst Rev.* 2017;1:CD005302.

8. Lin MG, et al. Misoprostol for labor induction in women with term premature rupture of membranes: a meta-analysis. *Obstet Gynecol.* 2005;106(3):593–601.

9. Amorosa JMH, et al. A randomized trial of Foley Bulb for Labor Induction in Premature Rupture of Membranes in Nulliparas (FLIP). *Am J Obstet Gynecol.* 2017;217(3):360 e1–360 e7.

10. Mackeen AD, et al. Foley plus oxytocin compared with oxytocin for induction after membrane rupture: a randomized controlled trial. *Obstet Gynecol.* 2018;131(1):4–11.

11. Committee on Practice Bulletins–Obstetrics. ACOG Practice Bulletin No. 188: prelabor rupture of membranes. *Obstet Gynecol.* 2018;131(1):e1–e14.

15

Antepartum Glucocorticoid Treatment for Prevention of the Respiratory Distress Syndrome in Premature Infants

MELISSA H. SPIEL AND JOHN ZUPANCIC

"[T]here is sufficient evidence of beneficial effects on lung function and of absence of adverse effects to justify further trials [with betamethasone]."
—GC LIGGINS ET AL.[1]

Research Question: What are the neonatal respiratory effects of a potent glucocorticoid given to mothers expected to deliver less than 37 weeks' gestation?

Funding: Medical Research Council of New Zealand

Year Study Began: 1969

Year Study Published: 1972

Study Location: New Zealand

Who Was Studied: Women admitted in premature labor between 24 to 36 weeks or in those for whom premature delivery before 37 weeks was planned.

Who Was Excluded: Those women for whom an obstetrician considered that corticosteroid treatment was contraindicated or those who delivered shortly after admission.

How Many Patients: 287

Study Overview: This was a randomized controlled trial. See Figure 15.1

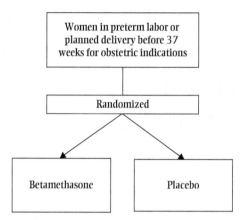

Figure 15.1. Study overview

Study Intervention: Patients randomized to the intervention group received a mixture of 6 mg of intramuscular betamethasone phosphate and 6 mg of betamethasone acetate or an identical appearing control with limited glucocorticoid potency. If undelivered 24 hours later, they received a second equivalent dose. Patients also received a trial of tocolysis for 48 to 72 hours using intravenous ethanol or salbutamol, unless membranes were ruptured, in which case the period was limited to 48 hours, as well as antibiotics. If delivery was planned for obstetric indications, the study drug was administered 72 hours prior to induction.

Follow-Up: First 7 days of life

Endpoints: Perinatal mortality, intraventricular hemorrhage, respiratory distress, Apgar scores, hyaline membrane disease, neonatal infection

---

RESULTS

- Infants delivered prematurely for premature labor (76%), hypertensive diseases of pregnancy (11%), Rh disease (7%), fetal malformation (5%), or placenta previa (0.7%).
- In the unplanned premature labor group, 226 infants were delivered. The rates of perinatal death (6.4% vs. 18.0%, $p = 0.02$) and respiratory distress (9.0% vs. 25.8%, $p = 0.003$) were significantly lower in the intervention

group, while the rate of intraventricular hemorrhage (5.3% vs. 0%, NS) was similar between the two groups.

- Among the participants who delivered after receiving full therapy (at least two treatments 24 hours apart) the rates of death and respiratory distress syndrome (RDS) were lower in patients who received betamethasone versus placebo (3.2% vs. 14.1%, $p = 0.02$; 4.3% vs. 24.0%, $p = 0.002$). The difference in RDS appeared to be driven by reduction of RDS in infants less than 32 weeks' gestation.
- A difference in rates of RDS between treatment groups was only seen in patients who delivered at least 24 hours after entry to the trial; it was not observed in patients who delivered less than 24 hours after entry to the trial.
- There were no antepartum or intrapartum complications attributable to corticosteroids.
- There was no significant difference between the groups in terms of neonatal fever within 14 days after delivery, lactation at discharge, or neonatal pneumonia.

Criticisms and Limitations: This study took place several decades ago, and although of generally sound methodology for the time, certain expectations of modern randomized controlled trials were not met. For example, no power calculation was provided, an issue of particular importance given the number of nonsignificant comparisons. Results were not provided for 21 women and their newborns, who were excluded after randomization.

The generalizability of the results is also an issue given very different practice styles in 1969. Older approaches to tocolysis (with a high proportion of delivery within 24 hours), treatment of preeclampsia or isoimmunization, and threshold for operative delivery might all affect the application of the results today.

Duration of follow-up was not explicitly stated but seems to have been limited to 7 days after delivery. Certain outcomes, including neonatal death, may have taken place after this time. Effect on longer-term neurodevelopmental outcomes was also not assessed.

The risk of neonatal death was higher in the betamethasone arm for mothers with severe hypertension, proteinuria, and fetal growth restriction. The reason for this is not clear.

Other Relevant Studies and Information:

- The premise of this study came from a basic observation by Liggins that lambs who had been exposed to antenatal corticosteroids in an experimental model of preterm labor had earlier lung maturation.[2]

- This first study was followed by a number of subsequent randomized trials of antenatal corticosteroids. By 1995, at least 18 trials had been completed, of which 15 reported clinical outcomes, in more than 3400 randomized patients. Meta-analysis of these trials suggested a strong treatment effect of glucocorticoids, with an odds ratio of 0.51 (95% confidence interval [CI] 0.42–0.61) for RDS and an odds ratio of 0.61 (95% CI 0.48–0.76) for mortality.[3] The most recent Cochrane collaboration meta-analysis now lists 30 randomized controlled trials involving 7774 mothers, confirming positive effects on perinatal and neonatal mortality, RDS, intraventricular hemorrhage, necrotizing enterocolitis, need for mechanical ventilation, and congenital infection.[4]

- Despite these compelling results, the adoption of antenatal corticosteroids in the United States was initially slow, with one estimate suggesting that by 1995, only 12% to 18% of preterm deliveries had been preceded by antenatal steroid administration. In 1995, a National Institutes of Health consensus panel reported its deliberations, with a strongly worded recommendation that "Antenatal corticosteroid therapy is indicated for women at risk of premature delivery with few exceptions."[5] Adoption in the ensuing two decades increased dramatically for pregnancies at risk of delivery before 34 weeks. Current American College of Obstetricians and Gynecologists guidelines recommend corticosteroid therapy for women at risk of delivery within 7 days between 24 and 34 weeks of gestation.[6]

- More recently, attention has been directed to the potential efficacy of antenatal corticosteroids in late preterm deliveries. The Antenatal Late Preterm Steroids (ALPS) study showed that infants of 34-0/7 weeks to 36-5/7 weeks gestation who were exposed to antenatal corticosteroids had reduction in composite respiratory support or mortality.[7]

Summary and Implications: This study demonstrated lower rates of perinatal mortality and RDS with administration of a course of antenatal corticosteroids in women delivering preterm. Based on this report and others, a single course of corticosteroids is now recommended in all situations in which singleton preterm delivery is anticipated between 24 and 33 6/7 weeks gestation, except when delivery is imminent. Corticosteroids may be considered for pregnant patients up to 36 6/7 weeks gestation.[5]

CLINICAL CASE: ROLE OF ANTENATAL STEROIDS IN WOMEN AT RISK FOR PRETERM BIRTH

Case History
A 25-year-old G1P0 presents at 28 weeks with preterm labor and is 3 centimeters dilated. Based on the results of this trial, how should this patient be treated?

Suggested Answer
A single course of corticosteroids is recommended for pregnant women at risk of preterm delivery, including those with ruptured membranes and multiple gestations. An attempt to delay delivery for 48 hours with tocolysis should be made, if not otherwise contraindicated, to allow for adequate time for corticosteroid benefit.

References

1. Liggins GC, Howie RN. A controlled trial of antepartum glucocorticoid treatment for prevention of the respiratory distress syndrome in premature infants. *Pediatrics.* 1972;50:515–525.
2. Liggins GC. Premature delivery of foetal lambs infused with glucocorticoids. *J Endocrinol.* 1969;45(4):515–523.
3. Sinclair JC. Meta-analysis of randomized controlled trials of antenatal corticosteroid for the prevention of respiratory distress syndrome: discussion. *Am J Obstet Gynecol.* 1995;173:199–206.
4. Roberts D, Brown J, Medley N, Dalziel SR. Antenatal corticosteroids for accelerating fetal lung maturation for women at risk of preterm birth. *Cochrane Database Sys Rev.* 2017;3:CD004454. doi:10.1002/14651858.CD004454.pub3
5. NIH Consensus Development Panel on the Effect of Corticosteroids for Fetal Maturation on Perinatal Outcomes. Effect of corticosteroids for fetal maturation on perinatal outcomes. *JAMA.* 1995;273(5):413–418.
6. Management of Preterm Labor, Interim Update. ACOG Practice Bulletin 171. Oct 2016, Reaffirmed 2018.
7. Gyamfi-Bannerman C, Thom EA, Blackwell SC, et al. Antenatal betamethasone for women at risk for late preterm delivery. *N Eng J Med.* 2016;374(14):1311–1320.

16

Outcomes Associated With Trial of Labor After Cesarean Delivery

HADI ERFANI AND ALIREZA A. SHAMSHIRSAZ

"Overall, our data suggest a risk of an adverse perinatal outcome at term among women with a previous cesarean delivery of approximately 1 in 2000 trials of labor (0.46 per 1000), a risk that is quantitatively small but greater than that associated with elective repeated cesarean delivery."

—MB LANDON ET AL.[1]

Research Question: What is the risk of uterine rupture and maternal and neonatal morbidity associated with trial of labor after cesarean delivery (TOLAC) compared with repeated elective cesarean delivery?

Funding: National Institute of Child Health and Human Development (NICHD)

Year Study Began: 1999

Year Study Published: 2004

Study Location: 19 academic medical centers belonging to the NICHD Maternal-Fetal Medicine Units Network

Who Was Studied: Women who had a prior cesarean delivery and who had a singleton pregnancy at 20 weeks or more of gestation or whose infant had a birth weight of at least 500g.

Who Was Excluded: Women presenting in early labor who subsequently underwent cesarean delivery.

How Many Patients: 45,988

Study Overview: See Figure 16.1 for a summary of the study design.

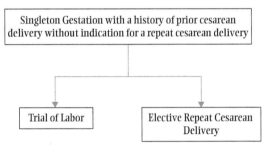

Figure 16.1 Study overview

Study Intervention: Outcomes were compared in this observational trial between patients who underwent a trial of labor and those who had a repeat cesarean delivery. Those who underwent a repeat cesarean delivery did so without labor but were candidates for a trial of labor, including those without a prior classical or "inverted T" incision, breech or transverse presentation, placenta previa, prior myomectomy, non-reassuring patterns in the antepartum fetal heart rate, or a medical condition precluding a trial of labor.

Follow-Up: Up to 120 days after delivery or the time of discharge for neonatal outcomes

Endpoints: Maternal adverse outcomes: A composite of uterine rupture, uterine dehiscence, hysterectomy, thromboembolic disease, transfusion, endometritis, and maternal death. Perinatal adverse outcomes: A composite of stillbirth, hypoxic-ischemic encephalopathy, and neonatal death.

RESULTS

- Women with a history of previous vaginal delivery were more likely to undergo a trial of labor. The overall success rate for vaginal delivery after cesarean delivery was 73.4%.
- The risk of hysterectomy, need for transfusion, and maternal morbidity are all statistically increased with a failed trial of labor compared to a successful vaginal birth after cesarean (VBAC), all $p < 0.001$.
- 124 cases of uterine rupture were reported in this study (0.7%). Among the cases with uterine rupture there were no stillbirths. There was a 1.8% incidence of neonatal death and 6.2% rate of hypoxic-ischemic encephalopathy.
- Maternal adverse events were more frequent with trial of labor (Table 16.1) and more common with an unsuccessful trial.
- Perinatal adverse outcomes were more common in trial of labor than elective repeated cesarean delivery (odds ratio 2.9; 95% confidence interval 1.7–4.8, $p < 0.001$); overall the risk of perinatal adverse outcomes is 1 in 2000 (0.46 per 1000) in a trial of labor after previous cesarean delivery.

Table 16.1. SUMMARY OF THE STUDY'S KEY FINDINGS

	TOLAC ($n = 17,898$)	Planned Repeat CD ($n = 15,801$)	Odds Ratio (95% CI)	*p*-value
Uterine Rupture, n (%)	124 (0.7)	0	—	<0.001
Hysterectomy, n (%)	41 (0.2)	47 (0.3)	0.77 (0.51–1.17)	0.22
Maternal Death, n (%)	3 (0.02)	7 (0.04))	0.38 (0.10–1.46)	0.21
Neonatal Death, n (%)	13 (0.08)	7 (0.05)	1.82 (0.73–4.57)	0.19
Overall Maternal Adverse Outcomes, n (%)	978 (5.5)	563 (3.6)	1.56 (1.41–1.74)	<0.001
Overall Perinatal Adverse Outcomes, n (%)	59 (0.38)	20 (0.13)	2.90 (1.74–4.81)	<0.001

Abbreviations: TOLAC, trial of labor after cesarean delivery; CD, caesarean delivery; ERCD, elective repeated cesarean delivery, CI, confidence interval.

Criticisms and Limitations: The primary shortcoming of this study is that it was observational, and confounding factors may have influenced the results. For example, women who opt to undergo a trial of labor vs. a cesarean section may differ in ways that might impact their outcomes. In addition, since this study took place at large academic centers, these findings may not be applicable to other lower resource settings.

Other Relevant Studies and Information:

- Prior to this study, a meta-analysis of 15 studies with a total of 47,682 women concluded that there might be a small increase in the rate of uterine rupture and fetal and neonatal mortality associated with TOLAC.[2] This meta-analysis also revealed a possible reduction in maternal morbidities including febrile morbidity, and the need for transfusion or hysterectomy in trial of labor.[2]
- A risk calculator has been developed to predict the probability of successful VBAC. This calculator takes the following variables into account: maternal age, height, weight, race and ethnicity, history of previous vaginal delivery, history of any vaginal delivery after the previous cesarean delivery, and arrest of dilation or descent as the indication for prior cesarean delivery.[3]
- A randomized trial examining psychological outcomes in women with a prior C-section who subsequently underwent a trial of labor versus repeat C-section found concluded that trial of labor can be offered and encouraged without concern for psychological morbidity associated with trial of labor.[4]
- In 2012, a prospective restricted cohort study concluded that among women with a prior cesarean delivery, a planned elective repeated cesarean delivery compared with trial of labor was associated with lower fetal and infant death or serious infant outcomes.[5]
- The 2017 American College of Obstetricians and Gynecologists Practice Bulletin on Vaginal Birth after Cesarean Delivery suggests that most women with one previous low-transverse cesarean section should be counseled about and offered TOLAC and emphasizes that prostaglandins should not be used for cervical ripening or labor induction in patients undergoing TOLAC.[6]

Summary and Implications: This study established the safety of TOLAC, demonstrating a VBAC success rate of 74% among women who undergo a TOLAC, and providing a relative risk of 0.7% uterine rupture rate among women who had a single prior cesarean section. Most women with one previous cesarean delivery with a low-transverse incision are candidates and should be counseled about and offered trial of labor.[6]

CLINICAL CASE: TRIAL OF LABOR VERSUS ELECTIVE REPEAT CESAREAN DELIVERY

Case History

A 32-year-old Caucasian G3P2002 with the estimated gestational age of 39 weeks and 3 days is being consulted regarding the mode of delivery. The fetal presentation at the first pregnancy was breech presentation, which required cesarean delivery with a low-transverse uterine incision. On the second pregnancy she experienced a successful trial of labor. Her BMI is 46. She is thinking about having another trial of labor.

How would you consult this woman?

Suggested Answer

Most women with one previous cesarean delivery with a low-transverse incision should be counseled that they are candidates for trial of labor. Based on the patient's history and the risk calculator for VBCD, the history of previous vaginal birth, especially when it is after the cesarean delivery, will increase the chance of having a successful vaginal delivery whereas the patient's BMI increases the risk of failure. The patient also should be counseled on 0.7% risk of uterine rupture, 0.2% risk of hysterectomy, and 0.02% risk of maternal death associated with trial of labor with a history of one prior low-transverse incision.[1]

References

1. Landon MB, Hauth JC, Leveno KJ, Spong CY, Leindecker S, Varner MW, et al. Maternal and perinatal outcomes associated with a trial of labor after prior cesarean delivery. *N Engl J Med.* 2004;351(25):2581–2589.
2. Mozurkewich EL, Hutton EK. Elective repeat cesarean delivery versus trial of labor: a meta-analysis of the literature from 1989 to 1999. *Am J Obstet Gynecol.* 2000;183(5):1187–1197.
3. Grobman WA, Lai Y, Landon MB, Spong CY, Leveno KJ, Rouse DJ, et al. Development of a nomogram for prediction of vaginal birth after cesarean delivery. *Obstet Gynecol.* 2007;109(4):806–812.
4. Law LW, Pang MW, Chung TK, Lao TT, Lee DT, Leung TY, et al. Randomised trial of assigned mode of delivery after a previous cesarean section—impact on maternal psychological dynamics. *J Maternal-Fetal Neonatal Med.* 2010;23(10):1106–1113.

5. Crowther CA, Dodd JM, Hiller JE, Haslam RR, Robinson JS. Planned vaginal birth or elective repeat caesarean: patient preference restricted cohort with nested randomised trial. *PLoS Med.* 2012;9(3):e1001192.

6. Practice Bulletin No. 184: vaginal birth after cesarean delivery. *Obstet Gynecol.* 2017;130(5):e217–e233.

17

Timing of Elective Repeat Cesarean Delivery at Term and Neonatal Outcomes

KATHERINE JOHNSON AND BRETT C. YOUNG

"Elective repeat cesarean delivery before 39 weeks of gestation is common and is associated with respiratory and other adverse neonatal outcomes."
—TN TITA ET AL.[1]

Research Question: What is the association between delivery before 39 weeks and the risk of neonatal adverse outcomes?

Funding: National Institute of Child Health and Human Development

Year Study Began: 1999

Year Study Published: 2009

Study Location: 19 sites across the United States (Maternal-Fetal Medicine Units Network)

Who Was Studied: Participants with viable singleton pregnancies delivered by scheduled, elective repeat cesarean section at or beyond 37 weeks gestation.

Who Was Excluded: Multiple gestations, a major congenital fetal anomaly, spontaneous labor, and medical or obstetrical conditions that warranted early-term or immediate delivery.

How Many Patients: 13,258

Study Overview: See Figure 17.1

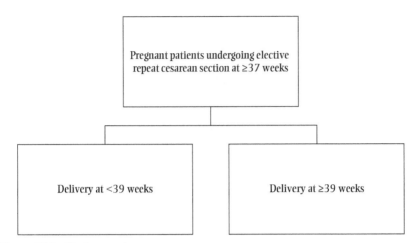

Figure 17.1. Study overview

Study Intervention: This was a prospective cohort study, evaluating the association of gestational age at delivery with adverse neonatal outcomes. Elective delivery prior to 39 weeks versus after 39 weeks was compared.

Follow-Up: Infants followed up until discharge from the hospital or 120 days after birth, whichever came first.

Endpoints: Primary outcome was a composite of neonatal death and several adverse events, including respiratory complications (i.e., respiratory distress syndrome or transient tachypnea of the newborn), hypoglycemia requiring treatment, newborn sepsis, and admission to the neonatal intensive care unit (ICU).

RESULTS

- In this multicenter study, more than one third of elective repeat cesarean deliveries were performed before 39.0 weeks.
- The primary outcome (neonatal death and severe adverse events) was less likely as gestational age at birth increased from 37 to 39 weeks. Several other neonatal adverse outcomes, including respiratory complications and admission to the neonatal ICU, were also increased at earlier gestational ages. These results are outlined in Table 17.1.

Table 17.1. INCIDENCE AND ODDS RATIOS FOR ADVERSE NEONATAL OUTCOMES ACCORDING TO COMPLETED WEEK OF GESTATION AT DELIVERY

Outcome	Week 37		Week 38		Week 39	
	%	OR (95%CI)	%	OR (95%CI)	%	OR (95%CI)
Any adverse outcome or death	15.3	2.1 (1.7–2.5)	11.0	1.5 (1.3–1.7)	8.0	Reference
Respiratory complications	8.2	2.5 (1.9–3.3)	5.5	1.7 (1.4–2.1)	3.4	Reference
Admission to NICU	12.8	2.3 (1.9–3.0)	8.1	1.5 (1.3–1.7)	5.9	Reference
Neonatal sepsis	7.0	2.9 (2.1–4.0)	4.0	1.7 (1.4–2.2)	2.5	Reference
Treated hypoglycemia	2.4	3.3 (1.9–5.7)	0.9	1.3 (0.8–2.0)	0.4	Reference
Hospitalization ≥5 days	9.1	2.7 (2.0–3.5)	5.7	1.8 (1.5–2.2)	3.6	Reference

Abbreviations: OR, odds ratio; CI, confidence interval; NICU, neonatal intensive care unit.

- Delivery at 41 and 42 weeks was associated with an increase in several complications.
- Attributable risk of the primary outcome due to elective delivery before 39.0 weeks of gestation was 48% at 37 weeks and 27% at 38 weeks, suggesting that that 48% and 27% of adverse outcomes could have been prevented by delaying these deliveries to 39 weeks.

Criticisms and Limitations: This analysis relied on accurate ascertainment of indication for delivery, which was derived from chart review. It is possible that an indication for earlier delivery was missed or miscoded. In particular, there was no information about decreased fetal movement, which could have prompted an early term delivery. In addition, the gestational ages of nearly a quarter of patients were potentially less accurate as they were dated by a third trimester ultrasound, which may confound the results. A sensitivity analysis, however, revealed that restricting the analysis just to those with dating by first or second trimester ultrasound demonstrated similar results as the overall cohort.

Some of the important adverse outcomes that could potentially be averted with earlier term delivery, such as stillbirth, could not be tested with this study design because this outcome occurs prior to the exposure (cesarean delivery). Other outcomes, such as neonatal death, are so rare that a difference by gestational age at delivery could not be detected with a study of this size.

Other Relevant Studies and Information:

- Elective delivery prior to 39 weeks is discouraged by the National Institute of Child Health and Human Development, Society for Maternal Fetal Medicine, and American College of Obstetricians and Gynecologists.[2]
- Infants born by cesarean delivery are at increased risk of adverse respiratory outcomes compared to those born by vaginal delivery.[3,4]
- Approximately 40% of 1.3 million cesarean deliveries performed annually in the United States are repeat procedures.[5,6]
- Analysis of primary cesarean sections has demonstrated an increased risk of adverse neonatal outcomes when performed prior to 39.0 weeks gestation.[7] Avoidance of elective early term deliveries is recommended regardless of mode of delivery.
- Elective early term delivery is not advised, but there is emerging evidence (the ARRIVE trial) that, among low-risk women, induction of labor at 39 weeks does not increase the risk of neonatal morbidity and may result in a lower rate of cesarean delivery.[8]

Summary and Implications: Elective delivery by repeat cesarean section is associated with worse neonatal outcomes when performed before 39 weeks gestation. Repeat cesarean delivery should not be performed before 39 to 40 weeks gestation unless there is a compelling indication.

CLINICAL CASE

Case History

A 30-year-old gravida 2 para 1 at 36 weeks gestation with a prior cesarean delivery for arrest of descent requests delivery by repeat cesarean. Her pregnancy has been uncomplicated. Her husband is in the military and will be deployed in 2 weeks; she would like a repeat cesarean section scheduled prior to his deployment. How do you counsel this patient about the risks associated with delivery prior to 39 weeks gestation? What are the absolute risks of an adverse neonatal outcome with elective repeat cesarean delivery at 37, 38, and 39 weeks gestation?

Suggested Answer

The patient should be counseled that elective repeat cesarean delivery prior to 39 weeks gestation is associated with an increased risk of neonatal morbidity including adverse respiratory outcomes, mechanical ventilation, admission to the neonatal ICU, hypoglycemia, newborn sepsis, and hospitalization for 5 days or more.

While the majority of infants born by elective repeat cesarean section will not have an adverse outcome, there is a 15% risk of adverse outcomes when an infant is born at 37 weeks and 11% when the infant is born at 38 weeks, compared to 8% if the infant is born at 39 weeks. These risks must be weighed against the benefit of timing the delivery for nonobstetrical indications.

References

1. Tita ATN, Landon MB, Spong CY, et al. Timing of elective repeat cesarean delivery at term and neonatal outcomes. *N Engl J Med.* 2009;360(2):111–120. doi:10.1056/NEJMoa0803267

2. ACOG Committee Opinion No. 764: Medically Indicated Late-Preterm and Early-Term Deliveries. *Obstet Gynecol.* 2019;133(2):e151–e155. doi:10.1097/AOG.0000000000003083

3. Zanardo V, Simbi KA, Vedovato S, Trevisanuto D. The influence of timing of elective cesarean section on neonatal resuscitation risk. *Pediatr Crit Care Med.* 2004;5(6):566–570. doi:10.1097/01.PCC.0000144702.16107.24

4. Annibale DJ, Hulsey TC, Wagner CL, Southgate WM. Comparative neonatal morbidity of abdominal and vaginal deliveries after uncomplicated pregnancies. *Arch Pediatr Adolesc Med.* 1995;149(8):862–867.

5. Martin J, Hamilton BE, Osterman MJK, Driscoll AK, Drake P. *Births: Final data for 2016.* Division of Vital Statistics; 2018. Retrieved from https://www.cdc.gov/nchs/data/nvsr/nvsr67/nvsr67_01.pdf. Accessed November 23, 2018.

6. Menacker F, Declercq E, Macdorman MF. Cesarean delivery: background, trends, and epidemiology. *Semin Perinatol.* 2006;30(5):235–241. doi:10.1053/j.semperi.2006.07.002

7. Hansen AK, Wisborg K, Uldbjerg N, Henriksen TB. Risk of respiratory morbidity in term infants delivered by elective caesarean section: cohort study. *BMJ.* 2008;336(7635):85–87. doi:10.1136/bmj.39405.539282.BE

8. Grobman WA, Rice MM, Reddy UM, et al. Labor induction versus expectant management in low-risk nulliparous women. *N Engl J Med.* 2018;379(6):513–523. doi:10.1056/NEJMoa1800566

18

The Natural History of the Normal First Stage of Labor

KARIN FOX

"The active phase of labor may not start until 5cm in multiparas and even later in nulliparas. A 2-hour threshold for diagnosing labor arrest may be too short before 6cm of dilatation, whereas a 4-hour limit may be too long after 6cm. Given that cervical dilatation accelerates as labor advances, a graduated approach based on levels of cervical dilatation to diagnose labor protraction and arrest is proposed."

—J Zhang[1]

Research Question: What is the natural history of normal labor of nulliparous and multiparous women?

Funding: Eunice Kennedy Shriver National Institute of Child Health and Human Development, National Institutes of Health

Year Study Began: 1959

Year Study Published: 2010

Study Location: The National Collaborative Perinatal Project was a databank from 12 hospitals in the United States, with prospective enrollment and data collection from 1959 to 1966.

Who Was Studied: A cohort of women, with normal, singleton, vertex pregnancies, who presented in spontaneous labor and delivered between 36 and 42 weeks

Who Was Excluded: Preterm deliveries or deliveries after 42 weeks, non-vertex, women with placenta previa, severe hypertension, cord prolapse, uterine rupture, neonatal APGAR score <7 at 5 minutes and those with less than 2 values of cervical dilation in the first stage and those whom did not becoming fully dilated

How Many Patients: 26,838

Study Overview: This study is a secondary analysis of prospectively collected data from a cohort database originally designed to study factors during pregnancy and early childhood, including abnormal labor progress, that affect child neurodevelopment and disorders such as cerebral palsy.

Study Analysis: Participants were grouped by parity and baseline characteristics were compared. Repeated-measures analysis with an eighth-degree polynomial model was used to construct average labor curves by parity.

The start time was set at the time in which the cervix reached 10cm, and labor time was calculated backwards. After the curves were calculated, time was reset to a positive value.

Because one cannot determine the exact time in which a cervix changes from one centimeter to the next (one only knows the time the change was identified,) the investigators used an interval censored regression to estimate the distribution of times for progression. The median and 95th percentiles were calculated for the curves.

For women in the cohort who contributed data from 2 or more pregnancies, a parametric frailty model was used to account for repeated measures from these participants.

Follow-Up: Women were followed until delivery.

RESULTS

- The overall cesarean rate in the National Collaborative Perinatal Project was 5.6%, with an induction rate of 7.1%. Twenty percent of nulliparas and 12% of multiparas had their labor augmented with oxytocin; 8% to 11% used regional analgesia.
- Approximately half of women in the cohort were White, 40% African American, 8% "other," mainly Latina, and a majority of women fell

between the 20th and 80th percentiles of the socioeconomic index based on data from 1960. Mean BMI was between 25 and 27, with an average weight gain of 10kg, and mean age was 20, 23, and 27 for parity of 0, 1, 2+ respectively.

- Median cervical dilation at admission was 3cm for nulliparas and 3.5cm for multiparas; mean gestational age was 39.8 weeks.
- All labor curves calculated in this study are exponential in shape, with the rate of dilatation accelerating as dilatation progresses in all parity groups. No deceleration phase was detected. See Figure 18.1.

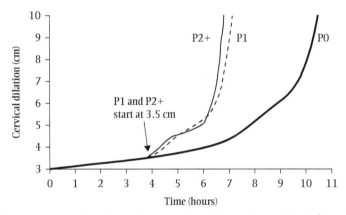

Figure 18.1. Zhang et al. The First Stage of Labor. Obstet Gynecol 2010 (published with permission).

- Nulliparous women had significantly slower labor progression and the most gradual labor curve; multiparous women of different parities had similar labor curves.
- The division between latent and active phases of labor was more obvious among multiparas than nulliparas, and no clear inflection point could be seen in the nulliparous curve, in contrast to the curve for multiparous women (with inflection points occurring at 5.5cm at parity = 1 and 5.0cm at parity = 2+).

Criticisms and Limitations: The study was performed using a database that is over 50 years old.[2-4] Practice patterns and patient characteristics have changed dramatically since the mid-20th century. The investigators, however, specifically chose to use this database, arguing that the current rate of obstetrical interventions, including induction of labor and cesarean delivery before the active phase of labor, introduces significant selection bias and limits the ability to study natural labor progression. Conversely, one could argue that the investigators' choice of dataset may no longer be generalizable to contemporary patients and practices, necessitating similar studies in the setting of today's patients and practices. The authors acknowledge these limitations in their discussion.

Other Relevant Studies and Information:

- Other studies have called into question the practice of using a threshold of 2 hours without cervical change, advocating for a 4-hour threshold with adequate contraction forces using an intrauterine pressure catheter, or 6-hour threshold without adequate contractions.[5-7]
- Studies assessing maternal and neonatal outcomes assessing the impact of extending the second stage of labor to prevent cesarean section have been published, almost all of which show a significant reduction in cesarean delivery rate.[8,9] Studies have mixed results regarding maternal and neonatal outcomes, with some showing no increase in immediate to short-term adverse outcomes. One large study showed that extending the second stage of labor led an increase in immediate adverse outcomes, such as the rate of shoulder dystocia, instrumental deliveries, and lower umbilical cord pH, but no increase in long-term adverse neonatal and early neurological outcomes.[10]
- The American College of Obstetricians and Gynecologists includes these reformulated labor curves in a consensus statement, "Safe Prevention of the Primary Cesarean Section."[11]

Summary and Implications: This study identified that the first stage of labor may be significantly longer than previously reported and that the rate of the second stage or "active phase" of labor varies significantly between nulliparous and multiparous patients.

CLINICAL CASE: NULLIPAROUS PATIENT PRESENTS WITH A VERTEX, SINGLETON PREGNANCY AT FULL-TERM IN EARLY LABOR (3CM DILATATION)

Case History
An 24-year-old G1P0 with an uncomplicated pregnancy presents to the labor and delivery unit at 39 weeks and 4 days with a complaint of frequent, painful contractions. On examination, she is dilated to 2cm, 80% effaced, at −3 station,

and is contracting every 4 minutes on tocodynamometry. She progresses spontaneously to 3cm dilatation over 3 hours while under observation and is admitted for labor management. After 2½ more hours, she is still only 4cm. After another hour, the cervix remains 4cm. The fetal heart tracing has been Category I throughout. Has her labor become protracted? What should be done next?

Suggested Answer

Traditionally, 3 to 4cm was considered the onset of the active phase of labor. Based on the study by Zhang et al.[1] active labor likely does not start until 5 to 6cm dilatation, and the onset of labor acceleration is more gradual in nulliparous patients. Provided there are no maternal or fetal indications, expectant management can be continued, as long as there is cervical change.

Had her cervical dilatation stalled, one could consider augmenting labor with oxytocin, and eventually assisted rupture of membranes once the head is well applied to the cervix. Using a 2- or 4-hour threshold for cervical change, this patient would be a candidate for intervention. Most experts would argue that considering cesarean delivery prior to any augmentation would be premature and contribute to an increase in the overall cesarean rate.

Suppose this patient remained unchanged for 3 hours at 9cm after augmentation of labor, rupture of membranes, with adequate force of contractions as determined by an intrauterine pressure catheter. Based on the findings by the investigators, the rate of cervical change should accelerate more quickly the more dilated the cervix, therefore waiting beyond 4 hours may be too long, and cesarean should be considered, rather than using a 4-hour limit.

References

1. Zhang J, Troendle J, Mikolajczyk, R et al. The first stage of labor. *Obstet Gynecol.* 2010;115:705–710.
2. Friedman E. The graphic analysis of labor. *Am J Obstet Gynecol.* 1954;68(6):1568–1575.
3. Friedman EA. Primigravid labor; a graphicostatistical analysis. *Obstet Gynecol.* 1955;6(6):567–589.
4. Friedman EA. Labor in multiparas; a graphicostatistical analysis. *Obstet Gynecol.* 1956;8(6):691–703.
5. Rouse DJ, Owen J, Hauth JC. Active-phase labor arrest: oxytocin augmentation for at least 4 hours. *Obstet Gynecol.* 1999;93(3):323–328.
6. Rouse DJ, Owen J, Hauth JC. Criteria for failed labor induction: prospective evaluation of a standardized protocol. *Obstet Gynecol.* 2000;96(5 Pt 1):671–677.
7. Rouse DJ, Owen J, Savage KG, Hauth JC. Active phase labor arrest: revisiting the 2-hour minimum. *Obstet Gynecol.* 2001;98(4):550–554.

8. Gimovsky AC, Berghella V. Randomized controlled trial of prolonged second stage: extending the time limit vs usual guidelines. *Am J Obstet Gynecol.* 2016;214(3):361.e361–366.

9. Rosenbloom JI, Stout MJ, Tuuli MG, et al. New labor management guidelines and changes in cesarean delivery patterns. *Am J Obstet Gynecol.* 2017;217(6):689.e681–689.e688.

10. Zipori Y, Grunwald O, Ginsberg Y, Beloosesky R, Weiner Z. The impact of extending the second stage of labor to prevent primary cesarean delivery on maternal and neonatal outcomes. *Am J Obstet Gynecol.* 2019;220(2):191.e191–191.e197.

11. American College of Obstetricians and Gynecologists (College); Society for Maternal-Fetal Medicine, Caughey AB, Cahill AG, Guise JM, Rouse DJ. Safe prevention of the primary cesarean delivery. *Am J Obstet Gynecol.* 2014;210(3):179–193. doi:10.1016/j.ajog.2014.01.026

19

Maternal Morbidity Associated With Multiple Repeat Cesarean Deliveries

MATTHEW K. JANSSEN AND STEVEN J. RALSTON

"Serious maternal morbidity increases with increasing number of cesarean deliveries. The majority of this risk is attributable to that associated with placenta accreta and/or the need for hysterectomy."

—RM SILVER ET AL.[1]

Research Question: Does maternal morbidity increase with an increasing number of repeat cesarean deliveries? Do placenta previa and placenta accreta contribute to that risk?

Funding: Supported by grants from the National Institute of Child Health and Human Development

Study Years: 1999–2002

Publication Year: 2006

Study Location: 19 U.S. academic medical centers as a part of the National Institute of Child health and Development Maternal-Fetal Medicine Units Network

Who Was Studied: Women undergoing non-labored cesarean delivery with pregnancy >20 weeks' gestation or with an infant birth weight of at least 500g.

All 4 years of the study enrolled women undergoing repeat cesarean deliveries and 2 years included women with primary cesarean deliveries

Who Was Excluded: Women with multiple gestations as well as those with cesarean sections preceded by labor, either primary or a failed trial of labor after previous cesarean

How Many Patients: 30,132

Study Overview: This was a prospective observational cohort study analyzing maternal and surgical complications of non-labor repeat cesarean deliveries in comparison to primary cesarean deliveries. See Figure 19.1. Obstetrical management and timing of delivery was left to provider and institutional standards. Trained research staff reviewed the logbook and database at each study center daily and were unblinded to number of cesarean deliveries. Data was collected through 6 weeks postpartum. Placenta accreta spectrum and postpartum endometritis were defined as clinical diagnoses except when histologic confirmation was possible in the event of hysterectomy. Cystotomy included a combination of elective and accidental cases whereas bowel injuries, ureteral injuries, and ileus were physician reported based on clinical suspicions.

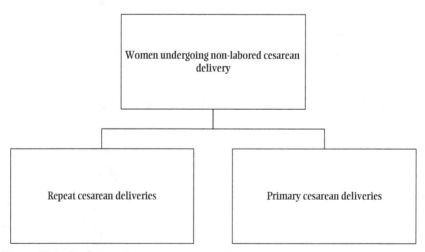

Figure 19.1. Study overview

Follow-Up: 6 weeks post-partum via medical records at the delivery institution

Endpoints: Primary outcome: Placenta accreta spectrum, placenta previa, bladder or bowel injury, peripartum hysterectomy, blood transfusion > 4 units, intensive care unit (ICU) admission, ventilator support, deep venous thrombosis, pulmonary embolism, postpartum endometritis, wound infection, wound dehiscence, ileus, and maternal death.

RESULTS

See Table 19.1.

- There were increased risks of placenta accreta, placenta previa, hysterectomy, blood transfusion >4 units, cystotomy, bowel and ureteral injury, ileus, ICU admission, ventilator assistance, operative time, and hospital length of stay with increasing number of cesarean deliveries.
- The majority of increased surgical morbidity with repeat cesarean deliveries was due to placenta accreta and peripartum hysterectomy.
- Patients with four or more cesarean deliveries experienced a 9- to 30-fold increase in the rate of placenta accreta and a 4- to 15-fold increase in the rate of hysterectomy.
- Patients with a history of cesarean section who were found to have a placenta previa had a dramatically increased risk for placenta accreta. The risk for placenta accreta was 3%, 11%, 40%, 61%, and 67% for first, second, third, fourth, and fifth or more repeat cesarean deliveries, respectively, with previa.

Table 19.1. SUMMARY OF STUDY FINDINGS

Number of Cesarean Deliveries (n)	Placenta Previa[a] % (n)	Placenta Accreta[b] % (n)	Risk of Accreta with Previa % (n)	Risk of Hysterectomy[b,c] % (n)
1 (6,201)	6.42 (398)	0.24 (15)	3.3 (13)	0.65 (40)
2 (15,808)	1.33 (211)	0.31 (49)	11 (23)	0.42 (67)
3 (6,324)	1.14 (72)	0.57 (36)	40 (29)	0.90 (57)
4 (1,452)	2.27 (33)	2.13 (31)	61 (20)	2.41 (35)
5 (258)	2.33 (6)	2.33 (6)	67 (4)	3.49 (9)
≥6 (89)	3.37 (3)	6.74 (6)	67 (2)	8.99 (8)

[a] *p*-value <0.001 after first cesarean delivery. [b] *p*-value <0.001 with increasing cesarean deliveries; associated with increased comorbidities of cystotomy, ureteral injury ventilator support, ICU admission, and reoperation. [c] *p*-value < 0.001 with increased comorbidity for pulmonary embolus.

Criticisms and Limitations: Some bias may be introduced from the relative homogeneity of the study centers. All cases were performed at academic medical centers, which may bias the findings toward increased morbidity given the large proportion of complex cases and resident training involvement. Conversely, these large tertiary care hospitals have increased blood bank and subspecialty resources, which may have mitigated some of the effects.

As placenta accreta "centers of excellence" develop along with other advances in management of placenta accreta spectrum such as uterine artery embolization and preoperative vascular balloon occlusion, the rate of modern maternal morbidity may be decreased compared to the reported data.[2,3]

This study focuses on maternal outcomes; a full understanding of the risks of multiple cesarean sections should also include neonatal outcomes.

Other Relevant Studies and Information:

- Subsequent studies also describe an increase in maternal and perinatal morbidity with subsequent cesarean section, particularly among women undergoing the third versus fourth cesarean delivery.[4,5]
- In 2014, the American College of Obstetricians and Gynecologists published a report "Safe Prevention of the Primary Cesarean Delivery" that aims to reduce the morbidities described in this study that result from repeat cesarean deliveries.[6]
- One trial reports increased cost-effectiveness of trial of labor after cesarean (TOLAC) versus elective repeat cesarean delivery, largely due to decreasing surgical morbidity related to placenta accreta.[7]

Summary and Implications: Maternal morbidity increases concordantly with the number of cesarean deliveries. Markedly elevated rates of placenta previa, placenta accreta spectrum, and peripartum hysterectomy with increasing cesarean deliveries seem to account for the majority of the associated morbidity. Overall, however, most repeat cesarean sections were uncomplicated, with few maternal deaths.

CLINICAL CASE: DELIVERY CHOICES—TRIAL OF LABOR VERSUS REPEAT CESAREAN

Case History

A 30-year-old G2P1001 presents for a routine prenatal visit at 28 weeks' gestation. The placenta is noted to be posterior. She has no medical or obstetric complications for the pregnancy. She has a history of a cesarean delivery for non-reassuring intrapartum fetal heart tones. She inquires about delivery options at your practice and states that she is interested in a repeat cesarean delivery although her sister is telling her to have a trial of labor. How do you counsel her on the effects of her delivery choice?

Suggested Answer

The current study provides important data that successive cesarean sections have increased surgical complications. Even though there are minimal concern for placenta accreta in this patient, overall morbidity is slightly elevated compared to her first pregnancy. It is also critical to have a discussion with the patient about future family planning. Although a cesarean section for this pregnancy may have minimal complications, if she is anticipating several more children after this, she may be facing significant morbidities with multiple cesarean deliveries. A desire for future pregnancies may be a reason to more firmly consider trial of labor. The data from this study can serve as an aid in this discussion, which should include consideration of the patient's values, intentions, and birth preferences.

References

1. Silver RM, et al. Maternal morbidity associated with multiple repeat cesarean deliveries. *Obstet Gynecol.* 2006;107(6):1226–1232.
2. Duan XH, Wang YL, Han XW, Chen ZM, Chu QJ, Wang L, Hai DD. Caesarean section combined with temporary aortic balloon occlusion followed by uterine artery embolisation for the management of placenta accreta. *Clin Radiol.* 2015;70(9):932–937.
3. Salim R, Chulski A, Romano S, Garmi G, Rudin M, Shalev E. Precesarean prophylactic balloon catheters for suspected placenta accreta: a randomized controlled trial. *Obstet Gynecol.* 2015;126(5):1022–1028.
4. Çintesun E, Al RA. The effect of increased number of cesarean on maternal and fetal outcomes. *Ginekol Polska.* 2017;88(11):613–619.
5. Gasim T, Al Jama FE, Rahman MS, Rahman J. Multiple repeat cesarean sections: operative difficulties, maternal complications and outcome. *J Repro Med.* 2013;58(7–8):312–318.
6. Caughey AB, et al. Safe prevention of the primary cesarean delivery. *Am J Obstet Gynecol.* 2014;210(3):179–193.
7. Gilbert SA, et al. Lifetime cost-effectiveness of trial of labor after cesarean in the United States. *Value in Health.* 2013;16(6):953–964.

First-Trimester or Second-Trimester Screening, or Both, for Down Syndrome

The FASTER Trial

JESSICA M. HART AND BARBARA M. O'BRIEN

> "Our results demonstrate that first-trimester screening for Down syndrome is highly effective, but combinations of measurements of markers from both the first and the second trimesters yield higher detection rates and lower false positive rates."
>
> —THE FASTER TRIAL RESEARCH GROUP[1]

Research Question: Should pregnant women be screened for the presence of Down syndrome in the fetus through first-trimester screening, second-trimester screening, or should measurements be incorporated from both trimesters for optimal screening results?

Funding: National Institutes of Health; National Institute of Child Health and Human Development

Year Study Began: 1999

Year Study Published: 2005

Study Location: 15 US sites

Who Was Studied: Women ≥16 years old who had a singleton pregnancy with a live fetus between 10 ³/₇ weeks and 13 ⁶/₇ weeks of gestation at time of study entry

Who Was Excluded: Women who had nuchal translucency (NT) measurements performed prior to study enrollment, a diagnosis of anencephaly in the fetus, or multiple gestations. Fetuses with findings of a septated cystic hygroma were followed as a separate subgroup.

How Many Patients: 38,033

Study Overview: See Figure 20.1

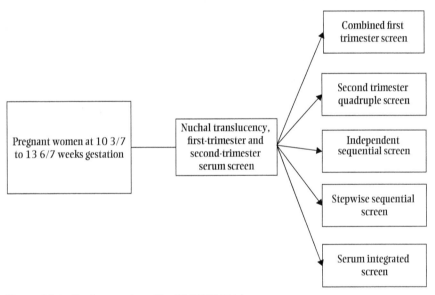

Figure 20.1. Study overview: The FASTER Trial

Ultrasound assessment of fetal NT was performed between 10 ³/₇ weeks and 13 ⁶/₇ weeks gestation. Serum markers were obtained at two points, once during the first-trimester between 10 ³/₇ weeks and 13 ⁶/₇ weeks gestation and once in the second-trimester between 15 ⁰/₇ weeks and 18 ⁶/₇ weeks gestation.

Study Intervention: First-trimester risk was calculated using measurements of the NT and two serum markers: pregnancy associated plasma protein A (PAPP-A) and the free beta subunit of human chorionic gonadotropin (fBhCG).

Second-trimester risk was calculated using measurements of serum alpha-fetoprotein (AFP), total human chorionic gonadotropin (hCG), unconjugated estriol, and inhibin A.

The following single trimester screening tests were evaluated:

- NT only.
- Serum screen only.
- Combined screen (NT and serum screening).
- Quadruple screen (AFP, total hCG, unconjugated estriol, inhibin A).

Sequential and integrated screening methods were also evaluated, including Independent Sequential Screen, Stepwise Sequential Screen, Serum Integrated Screen, and Fully Integrated Screen. See Table 20.1

Table 20.1. SCREENING TESTS FOR DOWN SYNDROME

Combined First Trimester Screen	First-trimester screen including nuchal translucency, PAPP-A, and B-hCG
Second Trimester Quadruple Screen	Second-trimester screen including alpha-fetoprotein, hCG, unconjugated estriol, and inhibin A
Independent Sequential Screen[a]	First-trimester combined screen followed by second-trimester quadruple screen. Second-trimester results calculated independent of first-trimester results/markers.
Stepwise Sequential Screen*	First-trimester combined screen followed by second-trimester quadruple markers. Second-trimester risk calculations incorporate markers measured in both trimesters.
Serum Integrated Screen	PAPP-A measured in the first-trimester, then second-trimester quadruple markers obtained. Second-trimester risk calculations incorporate quadruple markers with first-trimester PAPP-A.
Fully Integrated Screen	First-trimester NT and PAPP-A combined with second-trimester serum quadruple markers used to calculate a final second-trimester risk.

[a] Denotes results can be provided in the first trimester. Further results are available second trimester.

Abbreviations: PAPP-A, pregnancy associated plasma protein A; hCG, human chorionic gonadotropin.

Follow-Up: After all screening tests were performed, the patients were provided separate Down syndrome risk results from the first-trimester screening and from the second-trimester screening. Patients with a positive screening result were offered genetic counseling and diagnostic testing by amniocentesis if desired.

For fetuses with positive screening tests, suspected possible fetal or neonatal medical problems, and for a random sample of 10% of the enrolled participants, chromosome status was determined. This was done by (a) amniocentesis, (b) sampling neonatal cord blood if amniocentesis declined, or (c) tissue sampling if termination or spontaneous abortion occurred.

Endpoints: Detection rates and false positive rates for various Down syndrome screening tests.

RESULTS

- Combination screening tests, which include both first- and second-trimester markers, provided optimal screening performance for Down syndrome compared to single trimester tests.
- Better detection rates for Down syndrome were achieved with first-trimester combined screening at 11 weeks gestation compared to 13 weeks gestation, suggesting that the performance of PAPP-A and NT measurements declines with gestation.
- The performance of serum integrated screening is similar to the performance of first-trimester combined screening. Thus, if reliable NT measurements are not available, serum integrated screening is a reasonable alternative.
- Stepwise sequential screening has detection rates of Down syndrome similar to the fully integrated screening test.
- High detection rates of Down syndrome were demonstrated with the stepwise sequential screening test and the fully integrated screening test.
- Compared to alternative forms of screening, the fully integrated screening test yields the best detection rates and the lowest false positive rates. See Table 20.2.

Table 20.2. PERFORMANCE CHARACTERISTICS AND DIFFERENCES IN DETECTION RATES FOR PRENATAL SCREENING TESTS

SCREENING TESTS

5% FALSE POSITIVE RATE

	% False Positive Rate	% Detection Rate
Nuchal Translucency Only[a]	55	70
Serum Only[a]	42	70
Combined[a]	18	87
Serum Integrated[a]	15	88
Fully Integrated[a]	4.0	96
Quadruple	22	81
	% Points of Difference Between False Positive Rates	**% Points of Difference Between Detection Rates**
Serum Integrated vs. Combined[a]	−2.7	0.5
Fully Integrated vs. Combined	−14	8.6
Serum Integrated vs. Quadruple	−7.1	7.0
Fully Integrated[a] vs. Quadruple	−18	15
Fully Integrated[a] vs. Serum Integrated	−11	8.1

[a]The first-trimester markers were measured at 11 weeks' gestation.

Criticisms and Limitations: This study did not specifically address the rates of nonadherence to second trimester serum screening within the study population compared to reported rates in the literature. The American College of Obstetricians and Gynecologists reports that up to 25% of patients may be nonadherent with the second-trimester blood draw, which could significantly impact screening test results.[2]

In addition, a NT measurement that met quality control parameters could not be obtained in 7% of eligible study participants. Without the opportunity to perform quality assurance and to improve screening performance in these particular scans, these NT measurements may not have been optimal to detect Down syndrome. However, such quality assurance measures may not be available in all health care settings.

Other Relevant Studies and Information:

- Additional studies have demonstrated that combined first- and second-trimester screening tests (integrated, sequential, or contingent screening protocols) have higher aneuploidy detection rates compared to one-step screening tests.[2-4]
- Contingent screening, which was not evaluated in this study, has demonstrated detection rates comparable to the integrated and stepwise sequential screens, with the benefit that fewer patients were required to present for second-trimester lab evaluation.[5] Contingent screening involves first-trimester risk calculation by NT, PAPP-A, and fBhCG between 11 weeks to 13 weeks gestation. Low-risk screening results prompt no further follow-up, borderline risk results are recalculated using second-trimester data, and women with positive screen results are offered diagnostic testing.
- Noninvasive testing by cell free DNA (cfDNA) in the general obstetric population, when compared to standard aneuploidy screening including first-trimester combined, quadruple, serum integrated, fully integrated, or stepwise sequential screening, was found to have lower false positive rates and significantly higher positive predictive valves for detecting Down syndrome compared to standard screening.[6]

Summary and Implications: This large prospective study demonstrates that with appropriate quality control of ultrasound imaging, first-trimester combined screening for Down syndrome is effective. If first-trimester markers are unavailable, the second-trimester quadruple screen is a reasonable alternative. Optimal testing uses a combination of measurements from both the first and second trimesters to provide higher detection rates and lower false positive rates.

CLINICAL CASE: FIRST-TRIMESTER OR SECOND-TRIMESTER SCREENING, OR BOTH, FOR DOWN SYNDROME

Case History

A 25-year-old gravida 1 para 0 at 10 5/7 weeks gestation presents for her routine prenatal visit. She desires aneuploidy screening and discusses options with her prenatal provider. Based on the FASTER trial, how should this patient be counseled about her aneuploidy screening options?

Suggested Answer

The FASTER trial compared several strategies for detecting Down syndrome. Institutions will often simplify the screening algorithm based on known resources and baseline population risks, allowing practitioners to guide their patients through a smaller, select number of appropriate screening options.

In general, in a low-risk population, the fully integrated screen will likely be recommended as first-line screening as it provides a high detection rate and the lowest false positive rate of all the tests compared. The first-trimester combined screening test, which provides an earlier result, is also an effective option, although its detection rate and false positive rate are not as optimal. Stepwise sequential screening provides a first-trimester result and also has higher detection rates and lower false positive rates compared to single trimester screening. The serum integrated screen would provide the patient with effective aneuploidy screening if high-quality NT ultrasound measurements are not available. Lastly, with the advent of cfDNA patients should be aware of this screening option and be provided the necessary background on the strength and limitations of each screening test in making an informed decision.

References

1. Malone FD, Comstock CH, Dugoff L, Wolfe HM, Hackshaw AK, Lambert-Messerlian G. First-trimester or second-trimester screening, or both, for Down's syndrome. *N Engl J Med.* 2005:11.
2. Practice Bulletin: Screening for Fetal Aneuploidy. *Obstet Gynecol.* 2016;163. doi:10.1097/00006250-200305000-00052
3. Dugoff L, Society for Maternal-Fetal Medicine. First- and second-trimester maternal serum markers for aneuploidy and adverse obstetric outcomes. *Obstet Gynecol.* 2010;115(5):1052–1061. doi:10.1097/AOG.0b013e3181da93da
4. Baer RJ, Flessel MC, Jelliffe-Pawlowski LL, et al. Detection rates for aneuploidy by first-trimester and sequential screening. *Obstet Gynecol.* 2015;126(4):753–759. doi:10.1097/AOG.0000000000001040
5. Cuckle HS, Malone FD, Wright D, et al. Contingent screening for Down syndrome—results from the FaSTER trial. *Prenat Diagn.* 2008;28(2):89–94. doi:10.1002/pd.1913
6. Bianchi DW, Parker RL, Wentworth J, et al. DNA sequencing versus standard prenatal aneuploidy screening. http://dx.doi.org/10.1056/NEJMoa1311037. doi:10.1056/NEJMoa1311037

21

Cell-Free DNA Screening for Fetal Aneuploidy

The NEXT Trial

ASHLEY N. BATTARBEE AND NEETA L. VORA

"The performance of cfDNA testing was superior to that of traditional first trimester screening for the detection of trisomy 21 in a routine prenatal population."

—ME NORTON ET AL.[1]

Research Question: Does cell-free DNA screening for fetal trisomy perform better than standard screening among a routine prenatal population?

Funding: Ariosa Diagnostics and Perinatal Quality Foundation

Year Study Began: 2012

Year Study Published: 2015

Study Location: 35 centers in 6 countries including the United States, Canada, and Europe

Who Was Studied: Pregnant women at least 18 years of age who presented for fetal aneuploidy screening from 10 0/7 to 14 3/7 weeks of gestation

Who Was Excluded: Women with no standard screening result, known maternal aneuploidy or cancer, conception with use of donor oocytes, twin pregnancy, or empty gestational sac on ultrasound. Cell-free DNA samples were not included in the analyses if there was a low fraction of fetal cell-free DNA (<4%), inability to measure the fetal fraction, high variation in cell-free DNA counts, or laboratory assay failure. Additionally, women were excluded if they had a miscarriage, pregnancy termination, antepartum stillbirth, or delivered a neonate with a congenital anomaly suggestive of aneuploidy if no confirmatory genetic testing was performed.

How Many Patients: 18,955

Study Overview: See Figure 21.1

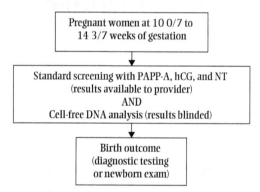

Figure 21.1. Summary of NEXT's Design

Study Intervention: All patients underwent standard screening with measurement of pregnancy-associated plasma protein A, total or free beta subunit of human chorionic gonadotropin, and nuchal translucency, the results of which were released to the provider. All patients also had cell-free DNA analysis, which was conducted in a blinded fashion with results not available to the patient or provider and clinical data other than maternal and gestational age not available to the laboratory personnel. Newborn outcomes were determined by medical-record review of the physical examination at birth and any prenatal or postnatal genetic testing. Outcomes were categorized as euploid or aneuploid and classified according to the type of abnormality.

Follow-Up: End of pregnancy

Endpoints: Primary outcome: Area under the receiver-operating-characteristic (ROC) curve (AUC) for trisomy 21 screening with cell-free DNA versus standard screening. Secondary outcomes: Performance of cell-free DNA for trisomies 18 and 13 with cell-free DNA versus standard screening. Performance of cell-free DNA for trisomy 21 in low-risk women (maternal age <35 years old or trisomy 21 risk <1 in 270 on standard screening).

RESULTS

- Among the 15,841 women who had standard screening and cell-free DNA analysis with neonatal outcome data, there were 68 chromosomal abnormalities (1 in 236). Of these, 38 were trisomy 21 (1 in 417).
- Cell-free DNA analysis had a higher AUC for trisomy 21, compared to standard screening (0.999 vs. 0.958, $p = 0.001$).
- Cell-free DNA analysis had better sensitivity (higher true positive rate), better specificity (higher true negative rate), lower false positive rate, and higher positive predictive value compared to standard screening for trisomy 21, 18, and 13 (Table 21.1).
- Among low-risk women, cell-free DNA analysis also had better test performance compared to standard screening. The positive predictive value of cell-free DNA analysis, however, was lower among low-risk women (76% for women <35 years old and 50% for women with trisomy 21 risk <1 in 270 on standard screening) compared to all women (80.9%).
- Compared to the overall study cohort, the prevalence of aneuploidy was higher among women excluded due to no result on cell-free DNA testing (1 in 38) and especially those with no result due to fetal fraction less than 4% (1 in 21).

Table 21.1. SUMMARY OF NEXT's KEY FINDINGS

	Trisomy 21		Trisomy 18		Trisomy 13	
	Standard Screening ($n = 15,841$)	Cell-Free DNA ($n = 15,841$)	Standard Screening ($n = 15,841$)	Cell-Free DNA ($n = 15,841$)	Standard Screening ($n = 11,185$)	Cell-free DNA ($n = 11,185$)
True positive	30	38	8	9	1	2
False positive	854	9	49	1	28	2
Trisomy	38	38	10	10	2	2
PPV	3.4%	80.9%	14.0%	90.0%	3.4%	50.0%
NPV	99.9%	100.0%	100.0%	100.0%	100.0%	100.0%

Abbreviations: PPV, positive predictive value, NPV, negative predictive value

Criticisms and Limitations: Calculation of cell-free DNA test performance did not include samples that did not pass laboratory quality control (i.e., those with a low fraction of fetal cell-free DNA), which would impact test performance. Failed cell-free DNA tests due to a low fetal fraction are associated with higher rates of trisomy 18 and 13 compared to successful tests; thus, genetic counseling and diagnostic testing are recommended in this setting.[2,3]

The authors were only able to compare cell-free DNA testing to standard first-trimester screening and not to integrated first- and second-trimester screening, which perform better. Furthermore, standard first-trimester screening can identify a wider range of abnormalities that cannot be detected by cell-free DNA analysis. Abnormal serum analyte screening may identify up to 17% of clinically significant chromosomal abnormalities other than the trisomy 21, 18, and 13 detected by cell-free DNA analysis.[4]

Other Relevant Studies and Information:

- Meta-analysis of cell-free DNA screening for fetal aneuploidy supports the findings of Norton et al.[5]
- Systematic review of cost-effectiveness of cell-free DNA for aneuploidy screening demonstrates that universal cell-free DNA screening is more effective but also costlier than standard screening with high incremental cost-effectiveness ratios.[6]
- The American College of Medical Genetics states that noninvasive prenatal screening with cell-free DNA can replace conventional screening across the maternal age spectrum, including low-risk women.[7] The American College of Obstetricians and Gynecologists (ACOG) and the Society for Maternal-Fetal Medicine (SMFM) emphasize that screening should be an informed patient choice with a foundation of shared decision-making, and in their most recent statement recommend that cell-free DNA screening be offered to all women regardless of risk.[8]
- Currently the National Society of Genetic Counselors still suggest that cell-free DNA screening not be used for "low-risk" women, although this is likely to be updated as the evidence evolves.[3]

Summary and Implications: Among a routine prenatal population, cell free-DNA analysis was superior to standard first-trimester screening for trisomy 21, 18, and 13. Cell-free DNA analysis was more sensitive with lower false positive rates, compared to standard screening. These data support the use of cell-free DNA screening for all pregnant women after discussion of limitations, benefits, and alternatives, as recommended before any type of genetic screening.

CLINICAL CASE: CELL FREE-DNA SCREENING FOR FETAL ANEUPLOIDY

Case History

A 26-year-old G2P1001 at 11 $^2/_7$ weeks gestation presents for her second pre-natal visit. She states that she heard there is a new blood test that can test for Down syndrome and tell her the sex of her baby. She wants to know more about this test and asks if she can get it today. Based on the results of NEXT, what should you tell her?

Suggested Answer

NEXT showed that cell-free DNA analysis is superior to standard first-trimester screening for detection of trisomy 21. It also appeared to be superior for detection of trisomy 18 and 13, although the study was not powered to assess these outcomes. However, cell-free DNA analysis is more costly than standard screening and cannot detect other abnormalities that may be recognized with standard screening.

The patient in this vignette should be counseled about the limitations, benefits, and alternatives of cell-free DNA screening as compared to standard first-trimester screening with serum analytes and nuchal translucency on ultrasound. The patient should understand that cell-free DNA screening will test for the common trisomies (21, 18, and 13), and if requested sex chromosome composition. She should be counseled that cfDNA screening has a higher detection rate and lower false-positive rate than traditional screening methods, but that cfDNA screening will only evaluate the chromosomes of interest, whereas traditional screening sometimes detects other abnormalities. Although detection rates with cfDNA are high, a normal result does not rule out these common trisomies. If cell-free DNA results are abnormal, genetic counseling and ultrasound are recommended to review further testing options. Diagnostic testing (amniocentesis or CVS) is recommended for abnormal results, similar to that after a positive first-trimester screen result. After informed consent, she may choose cell-free DNA analysis as a screening strategy.

References

1. Norton ME, Jacobsson B, Swamy GK, et al. Cell-free DNA analysis for noninvasive examination of trisomy. *N Engl J Med.* 2015;372(17):1589–1597.

2. Revello R, Sarno L, Ispas A, Akolekar R, Nicolaides KH. Screening for trisomies by cell-free DNA testing of maternal blood: consequences of a failed result. *Ultrasound Obstet Gynecol.* 2016;47:698–704.

3. Society for Maternal-Fetal Medicine Publications Committee. Consult Series 36: prenatal aneuploidy screening using cell-free DNA. *Am J Obstet Gynecol.* 2015;212:711–716.

4. Norton ME, Jelliffe-Pawlowski LL, Currier RJ. Chromosome abnormalities detected by current prenatal screening and noninvasive prenatal testing. *Obstet Gynecol.* 2014;124:979–986.

5. Gil MM, Accurti V, Santacruz B, Plana MN, Nicolaides KH. Analysis of cell-free DNA in maternal blood in screening for aneuploidies: updated meta-analysis. *Ultrasound Obstet Gynecol.* 2017;50(3):302–314.

6. García-Pérez L, Linertová R, Álvarez-de-la-Rosa M, et al. Cost-effectiveness of cell-free DNA in maternal blood testing for prenatal detection of trisomy 21, 18 and 13: a systematic review. *Eur J Heal Econ.* 2018;19(7):979–991.

7. Gregg AR, Skotko BG, Benkendorf JL, et al. Noninvasive prenatal screening for fetal aneuploidy, 2016 update: a position statement of the American College of Medical Genetics and Genomics. *Genet Med.* 2016;18(10):1056–1065.

8. Screening for fetal chromosomal abnormalities. ACOG Practice Bulletin No. 226. American College of Obstetricians and Gynecologists. *Obstet Gynecol.* 2020;136:e48–69.

22

Antepartum Assessment of Fetal Well-Being

The Biophysical Profile

JONATHAN S. HIRSHBERG AND NANDINI RAGHURAMAN

"Improved identification of the fetus at risk [for intrauterine demise] may be achieved when multiple fetal biophysical activities are evaluated [simultaneously]"

—FA MANNING ET AL.[1]

Research Question: Can antenatal testing that incorporates both ultrasound and fetal heart rate findings be used to decrease perinatal mortality in a high-risk pregnant population?

Study Years: 1980

Year Study Published: 1981

Study Location: University of Manitoba, Canada

Who Was Studied: Pregnant women at least 26 weeks in gestation with a pregnancy complicated by a "high-risk" feature. High-risk features included hypertension, diabetes, history of stillbirth, decreased fetal movement, restricted fetal growth, or pregnancies continued more than 2 weeks past the due date.

Who Was Excluded: Patients with uncomplicated pregnancies and lethal congenital anomalies

How Many Patients: 1,184

Study Overview: See Figure 21.1

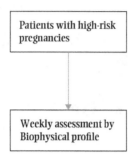

Figure 22.1. Study overview
*Twice weekly fetal assessment in patients with diabetes and postdates pregnancies.

Table 22.1. COMPONENTS OF THE BIOPHYSICAL PROFILE

Variable	Normal (2 points)	Abnormal (0 points)
Fetal reactivity	At least 2 fetal heart rate accelerations associated with fetal movement in a 40-minute period	Fewer than2 fetal heart rate accelerations in 40 minutes
FBM	The presence of at least 30 seconds of sustained FBM in 30 minutes of observation	No fetal breathing episode lasting at least 30 seconds in 30 minutes
Fetal movement	Three or more gross body movements in 30 minutes. Simultaneous limb and trunk movements are counted as a single movement	Two or fewer gross body movements in 30 minutes of observation
Fetal tone	At least 1 episode of motion of a limb from a position of flexion to extension and a rapid return to flexion	Fetus in a position of semi- or full-limb extension with no return to flexion with movement. Absence of fetal movement is counted as absent tone
Qualitative amniotic fluid volume	A pocket of amniotic fluid that measures at least 1cm in2 perpendicular planes	Largest pocket of amniotic fluid measures <1cm in 2 perpendicular planes

Abbreviation: FBM, fetal breathing movements.

Study Intervention: Trained perinatal nurses in two University of Manitoba teaching hospitals performed ultrasound and Doppler testing of the fetus. This testing, known as the biophysical profile (BPP) consisted of 5 components: ultrasound assessment of fetal breathing movements, fetal body movements, fetal tone, and amniotic fluid volume in combination with a fetal nonstress test. See Table 22.1. The fetus was assigned a score of 0 or 2 for each component for a maximum score of 10. This score was used to recommend a management plan for the pregnancy, from continued weekly testing for those with high scores (8–10) to immediate delivery for those with the lowest scores (0–2). Management of scores in the middle range (4–6) was dependent on fetal pulmonary maturity.

Follow-Up: Neonates were followed out to 28 days of life.

Endpoints: The primary endpoint used in this study was perinatal mortality (PNM), defined as death in utero of any fetus >500g, or death of a neonate within the first 28 days of life. The research team also collected data on any fetal anomalies detected during the BPPs.

RESULTS

- 1184 high-risk patients were recruited between 26 and 44 weeks' gestation and, as a group, they underwent 2,238 BPPs.
- The vast majority (97.3%) of the tests were scored in the normal range of 8 to 10, and only 0.35% of the BPPs were scored in the 0 to 2 range.
- The most common test characteristics to be scored as abnormal (0) were fetal breathing (72%) and NST (24%).
- Six perinatal deaths occurred in the entire study group (5 per 1000)
  - Four perinatal deaths occurred in patients with a BPP score ≥8, but 3 of these 4 cases were explained by other complications or inappropriate management that led to a perinatal death.
  - Two perinatal deaths occurred in patients with a BPP score ≤6, leading to a PNM rate of 42.6 per 1000.

Table 22.2. Observed Perinatal Mortality by BPP Score

	BPP Score Prior to Delivery ≥8 n (%)	BPP Score Prior to Delivery ≤6 n (%)
No perinatal mortality	1133 (99.6)	45 (95.7)
Perinatal mortality	4 (0.4)	2 (4.3)

Abbreviation: BPP, biophysical profile.

- Patients enrolled in this study had a significantly lower rate of PNM at 5.06 per 1000 than the predicted rate for a similar high-risk population of 65 per 1000, or the general population of low-risk pregnancies at 14.3 per 1000.[2] See Table 22.2.

Criticisms and Limitations: This study was designed as a prospective trial with only one study group. Patients all received the same testing and had standardized treatments based on the results of that testing. There was no control group with which to compare their outcomes. The authors instead chose to compare their PNM rates with the expected rates of PNM using normative data from the previous year. This limits any strong conclusions regarding the benefits of the proposed BPP intervention.

In addition, the study outcome was limited to perinatal mortality. There is no information provided on the other complications known to be associated with premature birth. This could be important as the BPP is a test that could lead to iatrogenic preterm delivery based on its interpretation. It is possible that performing this test may decrease the rate of mortality at the cost of more preterm deliveries.

Other Relevant Studies and Information:

- Manning et al. published a subsequent larger study 4 years later that included 12,620 high-risk pregnancies that confirmed the findings of this original trial.[3]
- A number of studies have been performed to determine the predictive value of the BPP. It has proven to be a reliable test of fetal well-being. In general, rates of perinatal death within one week of a reassuring BPP score (8–10) are extremely low.[4-6]
- The American College of Obstetricians and Gynecologists endorses antenatal testing (including BPP) in high-risk pregnancies while acknowledging that there is a lack of high-quality evidence from randomized trials that it decreases the risk of stillbirth.[7]
- The fetal non-stress test has also been shown to be an accurate method of fetal assessment when performed alone, with only slightly lower sensitivity and specificity than a complete BPP.[8]
- A "modified biophysical profile," which consists of the deepest vertical pocket of amniotic fluid and NST, has similar performance characteristics to the complete BPP.[9]

Summary and Implications: Based on this study, in high-risk pregnancies, the BPP appears to be an effective method of assessing fetal well-being, though the lack of a control group in the study limits the strength of the findings.

CLINICAL CASE: ANTEPARTUM ASSESSMENT OF FETAL WELL-BEING: THE BIOPHYSICAL PROFILE

Case History
A 33-year-old pregnant patient with Type 1 diabetes mellitus presents for late initiation of prenatal care. By last menstrual period dating, you approximate that she is 32 weeks in gestation. Her diabetes is currently managed with an insulin pump. Would you recommend antenatal testing for this patient? If so, what type and frequency of antenatal testing would you recommend?

Suggested Answer
Pregnant patients with Type 1 diabetes are at increased risk of adverse pregnancy outcomes including stillbirth, congenital anomalies, and neonatal morbidity. Identification of a compromised fetus in these patients may allow for appropriately timed intervention. The patient in this case is an example of a high-risk pregnancy included in the study conducted by Manning et al. In this study investigating biophysical profile testing in high-risk patients, the authors demonstrated a reduction in perinatal mortality when patients underwent biophysical profile testing compared to expected perinatal mortality rates in the regional population. This was one of the first studies to combine various individual parameters of fetal well-being, such as fetal breathing, tone, movement, heart rate reactivity and amniotic fluid volume into a single test.

The results of this study suggest that the patient in this case would benefit from twice-weekly biophysical profile testing. As mentioned in the study, this form of testing would also provide the additional advantage of identifying a potential congenital anomaly, particularly in a patient who has not received routine prenatal care.

References
1. Manning FA, et al. Fetal biophysical profile scoring: a prospective study in 1,184 high-risk patients. *Am J Obstet Gynecol.* 1981;140(3):289–294.

2. Morrison, I. *Annual report on perinatal mortality in Manitoba, Winnipeg.* College of Physicians and Surgeons of Manitoba; 1979.
3. Manning FA, et al. Fetal assessment based on fetal biophysical profile scoring: experience in 12,620 referred high-risk pregnancies. I. Perinatal mortality by frequency and etiology. *Am J Obstet Gynecol.* 1985;151(3):343–350.
4. Platt LD, et al. A prospective trial of the fetal biophysical profile versus the nonstress test in the management of high-risk pregnancies. *Am J Obstet Gynecol.* 1985;153(6):624–633.
5. Thacker SB, Berkelman, RL. Assessing the diagnostic accuracy and efficacy of selected antepartum fetal surveillance techniques. *Obstet Gynecol Surv.* 1986;41(3):121–141.
6. Vintzileos AM, et al. The fetal biophysical profile and its predictive value. *Obstet Gynecol.* 1983;62(3):271–278.
7. Practice Bulletin No. 145: antepartum fetal surveillance. *Obstet Gynecol.* 2014;124(1):182–192.
8. Devoe L., Castillo RA, Sherline DM. The nonstress test as a diagnostic test: a critical reappraisal. *Am J Obstet Gynecol.* 1985;152(8):1047–1053.
9. Miller DA, Rabello YA, Paul RH. The modified biophysical profile: antepartum testing in the 1990s. *Am J Obstet Gynecol.* 1996;174(3):812–817.

Diagnostic Tests for Evaluation of Stillbirth

STEPHANIE DUKHOVNY

"We conclude that placental pathologic examination and fetal autopsy are the most useful diagnostic tests for the evaluation of potential causes of stillbirth."

—STILLBIRTH COLLABORATIVE RESEARCH NETWORK[1]

Research Question: What is the usefulness of various diagnostic tests in the work-up for causes of stillbirth?

Funding: Eunice Kennedy Shriver National Institute of Child Health and Human Development

Study Years: 2006–2008

Year Study Published: 2017

Study Location: United States (all of Rhode Island and portions of Massachusetts, Georgia, Utah, and Texas)

Who Was Studied: All women delivering stillborn fetuses at or after 20 week gestation

Who Was Excluded: Deliveries resulting from termination of a live fetus

How Many Patients: 500

Study Overview: This was a secondary analysis of the Eunice Kennedy Shriver National Institute of Child Health and Human Development Stillbirth Collaborative Research Network Study. See Figure 23.1

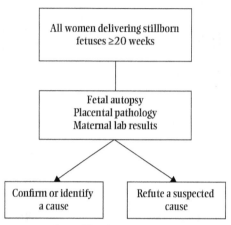

Figure 23.1. Study overview: the Stillbirth Research Collaborative Network

The purpose of this study was to assess the utility of diagnostic tests for the evaluation of stillbirth in a large, well-characterized, geographically, racially, and ethnically diverse population-based cohort. The study authors determined the "usefulness" of each diagnostic test, defined as a test that helped establish a probable or possible cause of death, or helped to exclude a cause of death that may have been suspected based on clinical history or other results.

RESULTS

- A probable cause of death was found in 60.9% of stillbirths.
- Overall, placenta pathology was the most useful diagnostic test, helping to exclude or establish a cause of death 64% of the time (95% confidence interval [CI] 57.9–72.0). Fetal autopsy was the second most useful test, yielding a useful result 42.4% of the time (95% CI 36.1–48.8).
- The following were the most useful tests stratified by clinical scenario:
  - Intrauterine Growth Restriction (IUGR): The most useful tests were placental pathology (88.7%) and fetal autopsy (79.2%). Antiphospholipid antibody was useful in 32.1% of those with IUGR.
  - Fetal anomalies: Fetal autopsy was the most useful test (90.3%); second was genetic testing (87.1%). Placenta pathology was helpful in 41.9% of these patients.

- Preterm labor, chorioamnionitis, preterm premature rupture of membranes: The most useful tests in this group were placenta pathology (80.5%) and fetal autopsy (44.2%).
- No clinical clues: The most useful tests in this group were placental pathology (78.3%), fetal autopsy (49.6%), genetic testing (13.9%), and antiophospholipid antibody testing (11.3%).

Criticisms and Limitations: Not all tests were performed on all stillbirths—not all patients consented to fetal autopsy, and not all serum blood tests were run at presentation. Results were obtained from stored maternal blood when possible.

Definition of a "useful" test was subject to determination by the study authors or by the classification system used. Ultimately, study authors took a practical approach to defining useful tests, taking into account accuracy, associated patient and system burdens, and the potential benefit of the test. Utility of some tests in practical application may also vary: for example, all pathologists in the study had undergone central training and followed a protocol. This may not be the case in all settings.

While the Stillbirth Collaborative Research Center is multicenter and population-based and represents regional and racial diversity, generalizability may be limited as the network was limited to 5 geographic areas, and the participating centers were largely academic centers. Counseling by the participating providers and general patient willingness to participate may also be different in this setting—for example, 86% of study patients consented to fetal autopsy; outside this setting the rate is closer to 50%.

Other Relevant Studies and Information:

- Other studies, including a large observation cohort from the Netherlands,[2] also evaluated tests and their utility in determining the causes of stillbirth; their findings generally affirm the results identified by the Stillbirth Collaborative. Placenta pathology and autopsy in particular are consistently to be the highest-yield diagnostic tests.
- The American College of Obstetricians and Gynecologists recommends fetal autopsy, placental pathology, and fetal karyotype as part of the testing in the setting of stillbirth. The maternal evaluation includes evaluation for fetal-maternal hemorrhage, antiphospholipid antibody screening, IgG and IgM for human parvovirus B-19, rapid plasma regain (RPR), and thyroid stimulating hormone (TSH). Thrombophilia evaluation is not generally recommended unless severe IUGR or personal/ family history of thromboembolic disease is present.[3]

Summary and Implications: This study is the first to stratify the utility of tests according to clinical scenario, providing the basis for clear, practical guidelines to evaluating stillbirth. In this cohort, placental pathology and fetal autopsy were the most useful diagnostic tests for evaluating cases of stillbirth. Genetic testing and screening with antiphospholipid antibodies were also useful in over 10% of stillbirths.

CLINICAL CASE

Case History

A 25-year-old G3P2002 at 24 weeks and 6 days presents with a fetus with severe IUGR. All measurements at the time of evaluation were <5%, and estimated fetal weight was 409g. Umbilical artery dopplers demonstrated persistent absent end diastolic flow. The fetal anatomy was limited but appeared to be normal. The placenta on the day of the ultrasound was noted to be cystic in appearance. The patient was otherwise healthy without major medical problems, although she did have mild range blood pressures on the day of her first ultrasound. Obstetric history was significant for 2 prior term vaginal deliveries, weights 5lb 12 oz and 6lb 6 oz. She was admitted to the hospital and counseled by Maternal Fetal Medicine and Neonatology. Amniocentesis was performed and chromosome microarray was sent, which demonstrated a normal female microarray. She received betamethasone, and her preeclampsia evaluation was performed and was negative, including a 24-hour urine protein. She was discharged from the hospital with close fetal monitoring. One week later, she presented with an intrauterine fetal demise at 26 weeks.

What workup should be offered to this patient?

Suggested Answer

This patient presented with severe IUGR. According to the results of this study, the most useful studies include placental pathology and autopsy. For this patient, placental pathology was sent and demonstrated a small for gestational age placenta with accelerated villous maturation and multiple remote infarctions, consistent with classic features of chronic placental insufficiency. She declined an autopsy. Antiphospholipid antibodies were also sent and were negative.

In this case, the placental pathology was revealing and demonstrated that placental insufficiency was the cause for stillbirth.

References

1. Page JM, et al. Diagnostic tests for evaluation of stillbirth: results from the Stillbirth Collaborative Research Network. *Obstet Gynecol.* 2017 Apr;129(4):699–706.
2. Stillbirth Collaborative Research Network Writing Group. Causes of death among stillbirths. *JAMA.* 2011;306:2459–2468.
3. Management of stillbirth. ACOG Practice Bulletin No. 102. American College of Obstetricians and Gynecologists. *Obstet Gynecol.* 2009;113:748–761.

24

An Intervention to Promote Breastfeeding

The PROBIT Study

LEANNA SUDHOF AND TONI GOLEN

"Not only is the Promotion of Breastfeeding Intervention Trial (PROBIT) the first randomized trial of the Baby-Friendly Hospital Initiative (BFHI) as a whole, but the large number of infants and mothers studied provides an opportunity to assess the direct relationship between a breastfeeding promotion intervention and infant health and the experimental link between infant feeding and infant morbidity in healthy mothers and their infants."

—MS KRAMER ET AL.[1]

Research Question: Does a breastfeeding promotion intervention result in a reduction of infant infections by affecting exclusivity and duration of breastfeeding?

Funding: Thrasher Research Fund, National Health Research and Development Program (Health Canada), UNICEF, and the European Regional Office of the World Health Organization

Year Study Began: 1996

Year Study Published: 2001

Study Location: 31 maternity hospitals and their associated polyclinics in Republic of Belarus

Who Was Studied: Patients with healthy term (≥37 weeks gestation) singleton births with a birth weight of ≥2500 g, an APGAR score of ≥5 at 5 minutes, who expressed the intention to breastfeed at admission to the post-partum ward, and whose infants were followed up at select polyclinics affiliated with the study site maternity hospitals.

Who Was Excluded: Patients who had contraindications to breastfeeding or conditions thought to interfere with breastfeeding; or patients not planning post-partum follow-up at a clinic associated with the study hospitals

How Many Participants: 17,046

Study Overview: This was a randomized controlled trial. See Figure 24.1

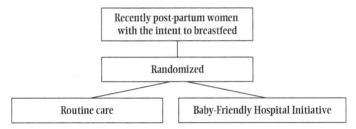

Figure 24.1. Study overview: the PROBIT Trial

Study Interventions: The intervention was modeled on the Baby-Friendly Hospital Initiative. The training of providers (nurses, midwives, obstetricians, pediatricians) at the hospitals and polyclinics took 12 to 16 months. The steering committee performed regular site visits.

Follow-Up: One year

Endpoint: Primary outcome: Risk of one or more gastrointestinal (GI) infections. Secondary outcomes: Risk of 2 or more respiratory tract infections, atopic eczema, recurrent wheezing, any breastfeeding at 3, 6, 9, or 12 months, and exclusive and predominant breastfeeding at 3 and 6 months. Exclusive breastfeeding was defined as receiving no solids or any liquids other than breastmilk; predominant breastfeeding was defined as receiving no solids or nonbreast milk (other liquids were permitted in this category).

RESULTS

- Patients in the intervention group had consistently higher rates of breastfeeding throughout the first year: at 3 months, 72.7% of intervention patients were breastfeeding (60.0% in the control group); by 12 months 19.7% of intervention patients were breastfeeding (11.4% in the control group). The odds ratios for having weaned at 3, 6, 9, and 12 months were 0.52, 0.52, 0.51, and 0.47 in the intervention group, meaning that the infants in the intervention group were consistently much less likely to have been weaned at any point post-partum in the first year.
- At 3 months, 51.9% of patients in the intervention group were predominantly breastfeeding; 43.3% were exclusively breastfeeding. In the control group, rates of predominant and exclusive breastfeeding were 28.3% and 6.4%, respectively. (See Table 24.1.)
- In the intervention group, infants had a 40% reduced risk of GI infection (9.1% vs. 13.2%) and a 46% reduced risk of atopic eczema (3.3% vs. 6.6%).
- There was no difference in infant respiratory infections between the 2 groups.
- The number of infant deaths due to sudden infant death syndrome (SIDS) was 1 in the intervention group and 5 in the control group.

Table 24.1. SUMMARY OF KEY FINDINGS

	3 Months		6 Months		9 Months		12 Months	
	I	C	I	C	I	C	I	C
Any BF	72.7%	60.0%	49.8%	36.1%	36.1%	24.4%	19.7%	11.4%
Predominant BF	51.9%	28.3%	10.6%	1.6%	NR	NR	NR	NR
Exclusive BF	43.3%	6.4%	7.9%	0.6%	NR	NR	NR	NR
Adjusted odds ratio of having been weaned (95% CI) [a*]	0.52 (0.40–0.69)		0.52 (0.39–0.71)		0.51 (0.36–0.73)		0.47 (0.32–0.69)	

Abbreviations: BF, breastfeeding; I, intervention; C, control; NR, not reported; CI, confidence interval.
[a] adjusted for birth weight, maternal age, and previous breastfeeding history

Criticisms and Limitations: In Belarus at the time of the study, formula was very costly, women had 3-year obligatory maternity leaves, and new mothers had post-partum inpatient stays of 6 to 7 days after a vaginal delivery. Furthermore, study participants only included patients who planned to breastfeed. This limits applicability to those who do not plan to breastfeed or who live in settings with different social pressures.

The study addressed the effects of breastfeeding promotion as an intervention, not of breastfeeding itself. Differences in clinical outcome may have also been attenuated by a relatively low rate of exclusive or predominant breastfeeding, as well as an unexpectedly low rate of GI infections in the first year (60% was expected; the actual rate was 19.7% and 11.4% in the intervention and control groups, respectively).

In addition, clinicians evaluating infants in follow-up were not blinded to the intervention; their assessments may have been altered by their knowledge of the intervention. This is evidenced by a report of falsification of trial data prompting an auditing of the records and the subsequent exclusion of the offending hospital from the study.

Finally, it is notable although rates of breastfeeding are significantly higher in the intervention group than the control group, rates of exclusive and predominant breastfeeding rates for intervention patients were only 8% and 11% at 6 months (for context, Healthy People 2020 objectives include a goal of 25.5% infants to be exclusively breastfed at 6 months). It is also notable, however, that the rate of any breastfeeding at 3 months was higher than expected in the control group, which suggests a general change in practitioner and patient awareness of the benefits of breastfeeding at the time of the trial.

Other Relevant Studies and Information:

- The benefits of breastfeeding are based mainly on observational data but include a reduction in severity and frequency of upper respiratory infections, GI infections, and atopic conditions in infants; a reduction in SIDS and infant mortality; a reduction in childhood inflammatory bowel disease, obesity, and diabetes; and a reduction in maternal rates of breast cancer, ovarian cancer, diabetes, hypertension, and heart disease.[2,3]
- The World Health Organization recommends exclusive breastfeeding for the first 6 months of age, with continued breastfeeding up to 2 years of age or beyond, and recommends instituting Baby-Friendly Initiatives to promote breastfeeding.[4]
- The US Preventive Services Task Force, American College of Obstetricians and Gynecologists, and American Academy of Pediatrics also recommend breastfeeding and breastfeeding promotion practices.[2,3,5]

- Several studies, including PROBIT II in which the children in PROBIT were evaluated at 6.5 years of age, suggest that children who were breastfed have a slightly higher IQ.[6–8]

Summary and Implications: Breastfeeding promotion can increase duration and degree of breastfeeding rates and may reduce the risk of infant infections in women who want to breastfeed.

CLINICAL CASE: PROMOTING BREASTFEEDING

Case History

A 28-year-old woman with a history of a premature delivery presents for prenatal care. On obtaining her history, you elicit that she had planned to breastfeed but never did because she was separated from her infant who was in the neonatal intensive care unit for many weeks. Due to her disappointment regarding her breastfeeding experience with that child, she does not want to address that issue during her pregnancy and says, "whatever happens, happens."

Suggested Answer

The PROBIT study demonstrates that women who receive lactation support are more likely to breastfeed exclusively or predominantly and are more likely to breastfeed for a longer period of time. This study also provides evidence of some of the clinical benefits of breastfeeding. The clinician should discuss recommendations for exclusive breastfeeding (1 to 2 years, with an initial 6 months of exclusive breastfeeding). Clinicians can reiterate both short- and long-term benefits for baby and mother. As support is a critical component of breastfeeding continuation, the clinician should be aware of existing supports—antepartum, within the hospital, and postpartum—and make them available to the patient. Hospitals can turn to the Baby-Friendly Hospital Initiative, which includes practices such as rooming-in, skin-to-skin contact, staff education, and a written infant feeding policy as a model for successful breastfeeding support.

References

1. Kramer MS, Chalmers B, Hodnett ED, et al. Promotion of Breastfeeding Intervention Trial (PROBIT). *JAMA*. 2001;285(4):413–420. http://ovidsp.ovid.com/ovidweb. cgi?T=JS&PAGE=reference&D=emed1b&NEWS=N&AN=6692221

2. American College of Obstetricians and Gynecologists. Optimizing support for breastfeeding as part of obstetric practice. ACOG Committee Opinion No. 756. *Obs Gynecol*. 2018;132:e187–e196.

3. American Academy of Pediatrics. Policy statement: Breastfeeding and the use of human milk. *Pediatrics*. 2012;129:e827–e841. doi:10.1542/peds.2011-3552

4. World Health Organization. *Implementation guidance: Protecting, promoting and supporting breastfeeding in facilities providing maternity and newborn services: the Revised Baby-Friendly Hospital Initiative*. Geneva, Swizerland; 2018.

5. US Preventive Services Task Force. Primary care interventions to support breastfeeding: US Preventive Services Task Force recommendation statement. *JAMA*. 2016;316(16):1688–1693. doi:10.1001/jama.2016.14697

6. Lucas A, Morley R, Cole TJ, Lister G, Leeson-Payne C. Breast milk and subsequent intelligence quotient in children born preterm. *Lancet*. 1992;339:261–264. doi:10.1016/0140-6736(92)91329-7

7. Kramer MS, Chalmers B, Hodnett ED, et al. Breastfeeding and child cognitive development. *JAMA Psychiatry*. 2008;65(5):578–584. doi:10.1111/j.1365-2214.2009.01070.x

8. Victora CG, Horta BL, de Mola CL, et al. Association between breastfeeding and intelligence, educational attainment, and income at 30 years of age: A prospective birth cohort study from Brazil. *Lancet Glob Heal*. 2015;3(4):199–205. doi:10.1016/S2214-109X(15)70002-1

25

Racial and Ethnic Disparities in Maternal Morbidity and Obstetric Care

ROSE L. MOLINA AND NEEL SHAH

"The present analysis . . . suggests that the racial and ethnic differences in maternal morbidities that were observed cannot easily be explained by differences in other patient characteristics or the hospital in which care was provided."

—WA GROBMAN ET AL.[1]

Research Question: What racial and ethnic disparities exist in obstetric care and adverse maternal outcomes?

Funding: Eunice Kennedy Shriver National Institute of Child Health and Human Development

Study Years: 2008–2011

Publication Year: 2015

Study Location: 25 medical centers of the Eunice Kennedy Shriver National Institute of Child Health and Human Development Maternal-Fetal Medicine Units (MFMU) Network

Who Was Studied: Women in the observational obstetric cohort for the Assessment of Perinatal Excellence (APEX) study

Who Was Excluded: Women who had no race or ethnicity recorded, or whose race and ethnicity was categorized as "other"

How Many Patients: 109,208

Study Overview: This was an observational cohort study of women who delivered in the 25 MFMU Network medical centers that were enrolled in the APEX study ($n = 115,502$). In this cohort, there were 6294 women who were excluded because they had missing data about race or ethnicity, or their race and ethnicity was categorized as "other." Therefore, a total of 109,208 obstetric patients with race and ethnicity recorded were included in the study.

Study Intervention: The investigators compared differences in maternal morbidity and obstetric care by the following racial/ethnic groups: non-Hispanic White, non-Hispanic Black, Hispanic, and Asian. They used multivariable models to control for demographic and historical characteristics as well as hospital of delivery.

Endpoints: Disparities in frequency of three maternal morbidities—severe postpartum hemorrhage (estimated blood loss ≥1500cc, blood transfusion, or hysterectomy for hemorrhage, placenta accreta, or atony), peripartum infection (chorioamnionitis, endometritis, wound cellulitis requiring antibiotics, wound reopened for fluid collection or infection, or wound dehiscence during the delivery hospitalization), and third- or fourth-degree perineal laceration—and disparities in specific obstetric care practices (e.g., induction of labor, episiotomy).

RESULTS

- The study population was 48% ($n = 52,040$) non-Hispanic White, 22% ($n = 23,878$) non-Hispanic Black, 25% ($n = 27,291$) Hispanic, and 5% ($n = 5,999$) Asian.
- There were multiple differences in demographic and clinical characteristics among the racial/ethnic groups.
- There were persistent differences in maternal morbidities by racial/ethnic groups even after controlling for patient characteristics and delivery hospital. Non-Hispanic Blacks, Hispanics, and Asians all had higher odds of postpartum hemorrhage and peripartum infection than Non-Hispanic Whites. Asians had two-fold increased odds of third- or fourth-degree lacerations compared to non-Hispanic Whites.

- There were persistent differences and variation in obstetric care by racial/ethnic groups even after controlling for patient characteristics and delivery hospital. Non-Hispanic Blacks, Hispanics, and Asians all had lower odds of labor induction than Non-Hispanic Whites. Asians had an increased odds of episiotomy while Non-Hispanic Blacks and Hispanics had a decreased odds of episiotomy compared to non-Hispanic Whites. (See Table 25.1.)

Table 25.1. SUMMARY OF KEY FINDINGS

	Non-Hispanic White	Non-Hispanic Black	Hispanic	Asian
Postpartum hemorrhage[a]	1.00 (ref)	1.71 (1.49–1.96)	1.51 (1.31–1.74)	1.54 (1.24–1.91)
Peripartum infection[a]	1.00 (ref)	1.25 (1.14–1.38)	1.45 (1.32–1.59)	1.62 (1.43–1.84)
Severe perineal laceration at SVD[a]	1.00 (ref)	0.76 (0.6--0.93)	0.86 (0.70–1.05)	2.06 (1.72–2.47)
Labor induction[b]	1.00 (ref)	0.88 (0.84–0.92)	0.67 (0.64–0.70)	0.74 (0.69–0.80)
Episiotomy[b]	1.00 (ref)	0.62 (0.56–0.68)	0.63 (0.58–0.70)	1.39 (1.26–1.54)

Data reported as odds ratio and (95% confidence interval)
[a]Adjusted for patient characteristics (age, diabetes mellitus, any hypertension, birthweight, prenatal care, obstetric history, multiple gestation, abruption, previa, accreta, anticoagulant use during pregnancy, insurance status) and hospital (fixed).
[b]Adjusted for patient characteristics (age, body mass index at delivery, diabetes mellitus, premature rupture of membranes or preterm premature rupture of membranes, cigarette use during pregnancy, gestational age at delivery, obstetric history, group B streptococcus status, insurance status) and hospital (fixed).

Criticisms and Limitations: While the study accounted for many possible confounders in the relationship between race and ethnicity and obstetric outcomes, it is possible that some relevant characteristics were not captured. Additionally, the study did not consider the roles of patient preferences in obstetric care or communication barriers that may have influenced some of the variation observed in different care practices among racial and ethnic groups.

Lastly, race and ethnicity are social constructs, and it is not clear how the categorizations of race and ethnicity were made (i.e., whether these were self-reported vs. assigned based on appearances). Native Americans were not included. Those who identify as multiracial and were categorized as "other" were not included as or were forced to choose one category, which leads to misclassification error.

Other Relevant Studies and Information:

- A study using the National Inpatient Sample from 2012–2015 similarly identified racial and ethnic disparities in overall severe maternal morbidity, blood transfusion, and hysterectomy with higher frequencies among all racial and ethnic minority groups.[2]
- A study done among New York City hospitals showed that hospital characteristics should be considered a significant contributor to racial disparities in maternal morbidity.[3]
- The American College of Obstetricians and Gynecologists and the Society for Maternal-Fetal Medicine have issued a committee opinion and special report, respectively, on racial and ethnic disparities.[4,5] Both reports highlight the drivers of and potential solutions for disparities at 3 levels: patient level, provider level, and health system level.
- The National Partnership for Maternal Safety convened multiple professional organizations to develop the Reduction of Peripartum Racial and Ethnic Disparities Patient Safety Bundle to address these disparities in perinatal outcomes at the hospital level (see https://safehealthcareforeverywoman. org/patient-safety-bundles/reduction-of-peripartum-racialethnic-disparities/).[6] Key components of the bundle include implicit bias training for the health care workforce and collecting, tracking, and reporting disparities for continual quality improvement.

Summary and Implications: This study demonstrated that racial and ethnic inequities exist in obstetric care and maternal morbidities after accounting for a variety of patient characteristics and hospital of delivery: non-Hispanic Blacks, Hispanics, and Asians experienced differences in rates of labor induction and had higher rates of complications of post-partum hemorrhage and peripartum infection than non-Hispanic Whites.

CLINICAL CASE

Case History

A 28-year-old primigravida at 39 weeks presented with pre-labor rupture of membranes. Her labor was augmented and she progressed to a vaginal birth with a second-degree laceration. She then developed a postpartum hemorrhage with an estimated blood loss of 1000cc and was found to have a fever of 101.1. She required a blood transfusion for symptomatic anemia. Your department quality assurance committee reviewed this patient's case because of the hemorrhage requiring a blood transfusion. A root-cause analysis revealed that there was a delay in admitting this patient to a labor room and a delay in starting oxytocin for augmentation of labor. There was no maternal temperature documented after admission. At the time of delivery, the patient's membranes had been ruptured for over 24 hours. Upon identification of the hemorrhage, the obstetrician and care team adhered to the hospital's postpartum hemorrhage protocol. The patient self-identified as Black with English primary language. What were the contributing factors to this patient's postpartum hemorrhage?

Suggested Answer

Addressing racial disparities requires a conscious effort to address the root causes of inequities, including social determinants of health and underlying structural racism. Within the health care system, OB/GYNs should make efforts to raise awareness of health disparities, to understand what community resources are available to women with limited access to health care, and to support quality improvement projects that target specific disparities within the health care system.

An explicit framework that includes race/ethnicity, language preference, and other social determinants of health should be applied to quality assurance and quality improvement processes. In the review of this case, it is important to include the patient's demographic information, and recommendations for improvement should consider factors related to patient demographics. In this case, it was determined that chorioamnionitis from prolonged rupture of membranes was a risk factor for postpartum hemorrhage. There was a discrepancy between what was documented in the nursing record and the physician record with regard to the patient's self-reported pain during early labor. Delays in admission and initiation of augmentation could have contributed to prolonged rupture of membranes. Maternal temperature was not recorded at the appropriate time points, which could have revealed signs of early infection. Labor floor acuity and care team implicit bias may have played a role in these delays. Steps to address disparity-related root causes identified during this review can include broader education regarding racial disparities in obstetrics, including discussions regarding implicit bias and its association with measured health outcomes.

References

1. Grobman WA, Bailit JL, Rice MM, et al. Racial and ethnic disparities in maternal morbidity and obstetric care. *Obstet Gynecol.* 2015;125(6):1460–1467.
2. Admon LK, Winkelman TNA, Zivin K, Terplan M, Mhyre JM, Dalton VK. Racial and ethnic disparities in the incidence of severe maternal morbidity in the United States, 2012–2015. *Obstet Gynecol.* 2018. Available from http://insights.ovid.com/crossref?an=00006250-900000000-97911
3. Howell EA, Egorova N, Balbierz A, Zeitlin J, Hebert PL. Site of delivery contribution to Black-White severe maternal morbidity disparity. *Am J Obstet Gynecol.* 2016;215(2):143–152.
4. ACOG. Committee Opinion: Racial and ethnic disparities in obstetrics and gynecology. *Obstet Gynecol.* 2016;128(654):1–4.
5. Jain JA, Temming LA, D'Alton ME, et al. SMFM special report: Putting the "M" back in MFM: Reducing racial and ethnic disparities in maternal morbidity and mortality: A call to action. *Am J Obstet Gynecol.* 2018;218(2):B9–B17.
6. Howell EA, Brown H, Brumley J, et al. Reduction of peripartum racial and ethnic disparities: A conceptual framework and maternal safety consensus bundle. *J Midwifery Women's Heal.* 2018;63(3):366–376.

The Risk of Pregnancy After Tubal Sterilization

Findings From the U.S. Collaborative Review of Sterilization the CREST Study

SUJATA CHOUINARD AND EVE ESPEY

"We found all methods of tubal sterilization to be highly effective in reducing the risk of pregnancy. However, the failure rates of most methods were substantially higher than those from most previous reports."
—HB PETERSON ET AL.[1]

Research Question: What is the risk of pregnancy after female sterilization with common methods of tubal occlusion?

Funding: National Institute of Child Health and Human Development

Study Years: 1978–1986

Publication Year: 1996

Study Location: 9 medical centers, mostly teaching hospitals, across the United States

Who Was Studied: Women who underwent tubal sterilization via laparoscopic unipolar coagulation, laparoscopic bipolar coagulation, laparoscopic silicone rubber band application, laparoscopic spring clip application, or partial salpingectomy by laparotomy (postpartum tubal ligation)

Who Was Excluded: Women who had a pregnancy, repeat sterilization, tubal anastomosis, hysterectomy, refused to be interviewed, or died

How Many Patients: 10,863

Study Intervention: This large prospective study, the U.S. Collaborative Review of Sterilization (CREST), was conducted by the Centers for Disease Control and Prevention and included 10,863 women undergoing different methods of tubal sterilization with long-term follow-up of 5 to 14 years. Nurses enrolled and interviewed women prior to the sterilization procedure and performed the annual follow-up contacts. Medical records were consulted for verification and details of pregnancies after sterilization failure. Survival analysis was performed using the life table method and Cox proportional hazards model.

Follow-Up: Annual telephone follow-up for 5 years with additional follow-up for up to 14 years for those enrolled early in the study

Endpoints: Primary outcome: Sterilization failure resulting in pregnancy

---

RESULTS

- 1.3% of women included in the study experienced true (method attributable) sterilization failure over the study period. The 10-year cumulative failure rate was 18.5 pregnancies per 1000 procedures. See Table 26.1.

Table 26.1. SUMMARY OF CREST RESULTS

Pregnancy Rates by Sterilization Method

	5-year (per 1000 procedures)	10-year (per 1000 procedures)	Ectopic (per 1000 procedures)
Postpartum partial salpingectomy	6.3	7.5	1.5
Silicone band methods	10	17.7	7.3
Bipolar coagulation	16.5	24.8	17.1
Spring clip	31.7	36.5	8.5

- 32.9% of pregnancies after sterilization were ectopic pregnancies.
- Postpartum tubal ligation with partial salpingectomy and laparoscopic unipolar coagulation had the lowest rate of failure (both 7.5 pregnancies

per 1000 procedures). The highest rate of failure occurred with laparoscopic spring clip application (36.5 pregnancies per 1000 procedures).

- Women under age 28 at the time of sterilization were at increased risk of failure compared to women aged 34 and older at the time of sterilization for all methods except postpartum partial salpingectomy. Increased fertility in younger women likely accounted for the difference.
- Black women were at significantly higher risk of sterilization failure compared with white women (relative risk 2.53, 95% confidence interval 1.59–4.02).

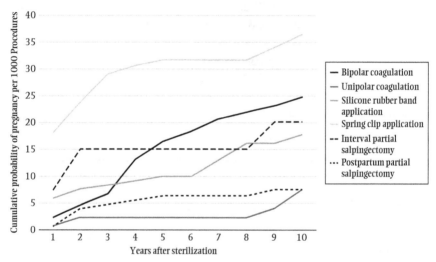

Figure 26.1. Summary of CREST results.
Reproduced with permission of MedReviews®, LLC. Bartz D, Greenberg JA. Sterilization in the United States. *Rev Obstet Gynecol.* 2008;1:23–32. All rights reserved.

Criticisms and Limitations: The study intentionally underestimated risk of sterilization failures by erring on the side of classifying pregnancies as luteal phase pregnancies (i.e., those pregnancies conceived before sterilization but only identified after the procedure, based on review of several data sources) as opposed to method-attributable failures.

The most likely source of bias is loss to follow-up; in particular, it is notable that young women and Black women were more likely than older or White women to be lost to follow-up.

The study population was not selected to represent the general population either in demographic characteristics or tubal sterilization method, limiting the ability to generalize the cumulative risk of sterilization.

Other Relevant Studies and Information:

- The spring clip (Hulka-Clemens clip) became less popular after publication of the CREST study; the more commonly, currently used titanium/silicone rubber clip (Filshie clip) appears effective.[2]
- A recently updated 2016 Cochrane review of tubal sterilization by the methods used in the CREST study found that all of these methods are generally safe and effective with few major complications.[3]
- Later analyses of the CREST database revealed a cumulative probability of expressing regret after tubal sterilization of 12.7%; risk factors included age <30 and undergoing sterilization postpartum.[4]
- The American College of Obstetricians and Gynecologists (ACOG) recommends comprehensive counseling regarding the efficacy, safety, and alternatives to female sterilization methods. ACOG further recommends that physicians discuss with all patients the risks and benefits of bilateral salpingectomy as a method of permanent contraception and vasectomy as a less-invasive and safer procedure than tubal sterilization.

Summary and Implications: This landmark prospective cohort study represents the most commonly referenced analysis of tubal sterilization failure rates. It demonstrated that tubal sterilization was less effective than previously thought and showed the increased risk of sterilization failure in younger women. Further, this study established that laparoscopic spring clip application, currently a lesser-used sterilization method, carried higher failure rates than other methods. These findings suggest the importance of accurate counseling about the risk of failure with each patient.

CLINICAL CASE

Case History

A Black 27-year-old G3P2 at 30 weeks gestation presents to the office for her prenatal appointment. During the appointment, she asks about birth control options following delivery, in particular permanent contraception. She states that she will have completed childbearing after this pregnancy. How do you counsel her about her options for permanent contraception postpartum? What are the risks of pregnancy following tubal sterilization for this patient?

Suggested Answer

CREST showed that young women (18–25 years old) were at higher risk of sterilization failure than older women. The patient should be informed about her higher risk of sterilization failure given her demographic characteristics and the high risk of ectopic pregnancy should she experience sterilization failure. She should also receive counseling about bilateral salpingectomy, vasectomy, and regret after tubal sterilization and other effective and reversible forms of contraception, including long-acting reversible contraceptives.

References

1. Peterson HB, Xia Z, Hughes JM, Wilcox LS, Tylor LR, Trussell J. The risk of pregnancy after tubal sterilization: findings from the U.S. Collaborative Review of Sterilization. *Am J Obstet Gynecol.* 1996;174:1161–1168.
2. Dominik R, Gates D, Sokal D, et al. Two randomized controlled trials comparing the Hulka and Filshie clips for tubal sterilization. *Contraception.* 2000;62(4)169–175.
3. Lawrie TA, Kulier R, Nardin JM. Techniques for the interruption of tubal patency for female sterilization. *Cochrane Database Sys Rev.* 2016;8:CD003034. doi:10.1002/14651858.CD003034.pub4.
4. Hillis SD, Marchbanks PA, Tylor LR, et al. Poststerilization regret: findings from the United States Collaborative Review of Sterilization. *Obstet Gynecol.* 1999;93:889–895.

27

Complications of First-Trimester Abortion

A Report of 170,000 Cases

MARYL SACKEIM AND SADIA HAIDER

"We conclude that outpatient abortion on selected patients to the 14th week from last menstrual period is a safe procedure."
—E. HAKIM-ELAHI ET AL.[1]

Research Question: Is outpatient abortion until the 14th week from last menstrual period (LMP) a safe procedure for healthy women?

Funding: Not documented

Year Study Began: 1971–1987

Year Study Published: 1990

Study Location: Three Planned Parenthood of New York City (PPNYC) sites

Who Was Studied: All patients undergoing pregnancy termination at 3 PPNYC sites were included. Between 1971 and 1978, patients included were at least 8 weeks pregnant by LMP. From 1978 to 1987, patients were required to be more than 5 weeks pregnant by LMP with a positive pregnancy test.

Who Was Excluded: Patients requiring in-hospital procedures, including those with a hematocrit <30, blood pressure of 160/110 mmHg or more, insulin-dependent diabetes, epilepsy, history of a bleeding disorder, or acute cardiopulmonary disease were excluded. Patients not fasting upon presentation, those who had a clinically suspected sexually transmitted disease (STD) or required preoperative antibiotics were also excluded. In 1979, when general anesthesia was made available at one site, other exclusion criteria were added including contraindications to methohexital anesthesia, history of sensitivity to barbiturates, presence of porphyria, and morbid obesity.

How Many Patients: 170,000

Study Overview: This is a retrospective cohort study evaluating outcomes of 170,000 abortions performed at three outpatient clinics from 1971–1987. Ultrasound was used to assist in determining gestational age only if there was uncertainty based on LMP and exam. Physicians performed all procedures under the same "standards and guidelines,"[1] including using a modified sterile technique, a single-tooth tenaculum to grasp the cervix, Pratt dilators for cervical dilation, and a combination of suction and sharp curettage for uterine evacuation. Ergotrate maleate was given post-procedure for increased bleeding or for history of hemorrhage. The specimen was examined grossly, and all tissue was submitted to pathology. If no fetal tissue was obtained, patients were referred to hospitals to rule out an ectopic pregnancy. Patients had the option of receiving a post-abortal intrauterine device (IUD) until 1985. No routine pre- or post-procedure antibiotics were given.

Follow-Up: 2 to 3 weeks

Endpoints: Deaths, major complications requiring hospitalization (sepsis, uterine perforation, vaginal bleeding, inability to complete abortion, incomplete abortion, heterotopic pregnancy), and minor complications requiring outpatient treatment (mild infection, repeat suction on day of surgery or subsequently, cervical stenosis or tear, underestimation of gestational age, seizure)

RESULTS

- Among 170,000 first trimester abortions, there were no deaths noted.
- 1 in 1405 (0.071%) patients experienced a major complication requiring hospitalization (Table 27.1). Incomplete abortion was the most common complication with a rate of 0.028% ($n = 47$). The rate of uterine perforation was notably low (0.009%). There was no recognized organ damage. There were no subsequent hysterectomies.

- 1 in 118 (0.846%) patients experienced a minor complication rate that required outpatient treatment (Table 27.1). The most common minor complication was mild infection (0.46%). Post-procedure, 37 patients were found to have an ectopic pregnancy and, of those, 4 were heterotopic.
- 58 patients did not get a procedure due to concern for ectopic pregnancy. Rates of complications were similar for patients whether they received general or local anesthesia.
- Cervical preparation was not used in the standardized protocols. The study demonstrated low rates of uterine perforation or cervical injury.

Table 27.1. COMPLICATIONS OF FIRST-TRIMESTER ABORTION REQUIRING HOSPITALIZATION

	Number of Cases	Occurrence Rate
Major Complications	121 (0.071%)	1 in 1405
Incomplete abortion[a]	47 (0.028%)	1 in 3617
Sepsis[b]	36 (0.021%)	1 in 4722
Minor Complications	1438 (0.846%)	1 in 118
Mild infection	784 (0.46%)	1 in 216
Resuctioned day of surgery	307 (0.18%)	1 in 553
Resuctioned subsequently	285 (0.17%)	1 in 596

Note: Cervical stenosis, cervical tear, uterine perforation, vaginal bleeding requiring hospitalization, and inability to complete abortion each occurred at rates of less than 1 in 5000.
[a]Requiring repeat curettage in hospital. [b]Defined as 2 or more days of fever 40C or higher.

Criticisms and Limitations: The observational study design is limited by loss-to-follow-up, which was 8% ($n = 1360$). Some of these patients may have had complications treated elsewhere that were not included as outcomes; therefore, the results are biased toward underreporting.

Reported complication rates were categorized differently than the standard CDC classifications and were lower than those published previously, including multiple studies of first-trimester abortion complications that incorporate CDC data.[2] The ectopic pregnancy rate was low at 0.056% ($n = 95$), lower than the ectopic pregnancy rate reported by the CDC of 2% of all reported pregnancies,[3] potentially because most procedures occurred after 8 weeks gestation. Cervical stenosis was 0.028% ($n = 28$), possibly due to the routine use of sharp curettage.

Finally, length of procedure, patient discomfort, and patient or provider satisfaction were not assessed.

Other Relevant Studies and Information: New York legalized abortion in 1970, 3 years before the *Roe vs. Wade* Supreme Court decision. From 1971 to 1972, Planned Parenthood opened 3 abortion sites in New York City as a low-cost, outpatient alternative to hospital-based abortion, most of which was performed under general anesthesia. Previous studies reported on the safety of abortion up to 12 weeks gestation and were limited by "a wide range of variance"[1] in study design and clinic protocols. This study uniquely captured a large patient population within a single organization with uniform protocols up to 14 weeks gestation, demonstrating the safety of outpatient abortions.

The low rate of complications in 1st trimester abortion has been confirmed in more recent studies[4,5] and has demonstrated safety for patients with chronic medical problems.[5] The greater prevalence of obesity presents a potential challenge, but abortion complication rates overall do not appear to be increased for obese women in the first trimester.[5,6] Recent literature has also demonstrated the safety of moderate intravenous sedation for obese patients undergoing first-trimester surgical abortion.[7]

The standard for dilation and curettage described in this study (rigid dilators, suction cannula, sharp curettage, and final aspiration) has undergone little change since 1990. However, sharp curettage is no longer routinely used, and routine antibiotic prophylaxis is now recommended for all women undergoing surgical abortion (study patients did not routinely receive pre-procedure antibiotics).[8,9]

Summary and Implications: This study establishes that dilation and curettage for first-trimester abortion can be safely performed in the ambulatory setting, without advanced cervical preparation, and under either local or general anesthesia. Rates of complication among these patients were low. Because of this and other studies, the American College of Obstetricians and Gynecologists has affirmed "safe, legal abortion as a necessary component off women's health care."[10]

CLINICAL CASE

Case History

A 28-year-old woman presents for STD testing after unprotected sex, is found to be pregnant, and desires termination. Vital signs are normal. Physical exam is notable for a BMI of 37. Hemoglobin is 11.5. Blood type is O+. Cervical cultures are collected. An ultrasound confirms a gestational age of 12 weeks 2 days. She desires an IUD for contraception. Based on the results of this study, can this patient safely undergo an outpatient surgical abortion?

Suggested Answer

This patient can safely undergo outpatient surgical abortion with a very low probability of complications under local anesthesia, moderate sedation, or general anesthesia. As demonstrated in subsequent studies, she should receive prophylactic antibiotics prior to her procedure, and an immediate post-abortion IUD can be placed safely.

References

1. Hakim-Elahi E, Tovell HM, Burnhill MS. Complications of first-trimester abortion: a report of 170,000 cases. *Obstet Gynecol.* 1990;76(1):129–135.
2. Cates WaG, D. Morbidity and mortality of abortion in the United States. In: *Abortion and Sterilization: Medical and Social Aspects.* London: Academic Press; 1981:155–180.
3. Ectopic pregnancy--United States, 1990–1992. *MMWR.* 1995;44(3):46–48.
4. White K, Carroll E, Grossman D. Complications from first-trimester aspiration abortion: a systematic review of the literature. *Contraception.* 2015;92(5):422–438.
5. Guiahi M, Schiller G, Sheeder J, Teal S. Safety of first-trimester uterine evacuation in the outpatient setting for women with common chronic conditions. *Contraception.* 2015;92(5):453–457.
6. Benson LS, Micks EA, Ingalls C, Prager SW. Safety of outpatient surgical abortion for obese patients in the first and second trimesters. *Obstet Gynecol.* 2016;128(5):1065–1070.
7. Horwitz G, Roncari D, Braaten KP, Maurer R, Fortin J, Goldberg AB. Moderate intravenous sedation for first trimester surgical abortion: a comparison of adverse outcomes between obese and normal-weight women. *Contraception.* 2018;97(1):48–53.
8. Sawaya GF, Grady D, Kerlikowske K, Grimes DA. Antibiotics at the time of induced abortion: the case for universal prophylaxis based on a meta-analysis. *Obstet Gynecol.* 1996;87(5 Pt 2):884–890.
9. Low N, Mueller M, Van Vliet HA, Kapp N. Perioperative antibiotics to prevent infection after first-trimester abortion. *Cochrane Database Sys Rev.* 2012(3):Cd005217.
10. Committee on Health Care for Underserved Women. ACOG Committee Opinion No. 613: increasing access to abortion. *Obstet Gynecol.* 2014;124(5):1060–1065. doi:10.1097/01.AOG.0000456326.88857.31

28

Long-Acting Reversible Contraception Versus Pills/Patch/Ring

The Contraceptive CHOICE Project

ANTOINETTE DANVERS AND ELIZABETH B. SCHMIDT

"The effectiveness of long-acting reversible contraception is superior to that of contraceptive pills, patch, or ring and is not altered in adolescents and young women."
—B WINNER ET AL.[1]

Research Question: What are the rates of contraceptive failure of intrauterine devices (IUDs) and contraceptive implants versus commonly prescribed contraceptives?

Funding: Susan Thompson Buffet Foundation

Year Study Began: 2007–2011

Year Study Published: 2012

Study Location: St. Louis, Missouri

Who Was Studied: Sexually active women between the ages 14 to 45 at risk for pregnancy who were seeking to switch or start a new contraceptive method. All participants stated a desire to not become pregnant for at least the next 12 months.

Who Was Excluded: Women who had undergone hysterectomy or sterilization were excluded from participation in the study. Participants who were intermittently using condoms, diaphragm, and natural family planning were excluded from the analysis.

How Many Patients: 7,486

Study Overview: See Figure 28.1

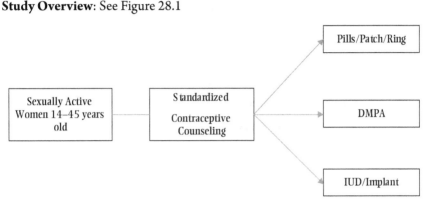

Figure 28.1. Study overview: the contraceptive CHOICE Project

Study Intervention: This was a prospective cohort study. Women were screened for eligibility at which time they received a scripted overview of all long-acting reversible contraception (LARC) methods. Those participants eligible for enrollment received contraception counseling for all reversible methods before informed consent was obtained. Participants then received the contraceptive method of their choice at no cost. They were able to switch to a different method during the 2-to 3-year follow-up period.

Follow-Up: Telephone interviews at 3 and 6 months, then every 6 months.

Endpoints: Primary outcome: Contraceptive failure resulting in unintended pregnancy. Secondary outcome: Pregnancy rates by age group

RESULTS

- Among 7486 patients there were 334 unintended pregnancies; 156 were attributed to contraceptive failure.
- Patients using the pill/patch/ring were 21.8 times more likely to experience an unintended pregnancy than with use of IUD or implants (hazard ratio = 21.8; 95% confidence interval 13.7–34.9).

- In years 1, 2, and 3 of the study, failure rates among pill/patch/ring users were higher than those using IUD or implant (p <0.001) (Table 28.1). Risks of unintended pregnancy among pill/patch/ring users were significantly higher (4.55 per 100 participants) than in those who used IUD or implants (0.27 per 100 participants).
- Failure rates among the group using depo medroxyprogesterone acetate (DMPA) injection were similar to those using IUDs or implant. Women less than 21 years of age who were using pills/patch/ring were almost twice as likely to experience an unintended pregnancy as women over the age of 21 using the same method.

Table 28.1. SUMMARY OF KEY STUDY FINDINGS: CUMULATIVE PERCENTAGE OF CONTRACEPTIVE FAILURE AT 1, 2, AND 3 YEARS

	IUD/Implant	DMPA	Pill/Patch/Ring
Year 1	0.3	0.1	4.8
Year 2	0.6	0.7	7.8
Year 3	0.9	0.7	9.4

Number of pregnancies attributed to IUD, implant, DMPA, pill, patch, or ring failure was 156. Participants using pill, patch or ring had significantly more unintended pregnancies than those using LARC (p <0.001) or DMPA (p <0.001).
Abbreviations: IUD, intrauterine device; DMPA, depo medroxyprogesterone acetate; LARC, long-acting reversible contraception.

Criticisms and Limitations: The trial targeted women that were at high risk for unintended pregnancy who were willing to switch to a new method, which limits the study's generalizability. The uptake of LARC devices was >70%, which was significantly higher than that of the general population.[2] The increase in uptake is thought to be secondary to the provision of no-cost contraception, but it is unclear what impact population characteristics have on participants' decision to choose LARC compared to the general population. In addition, the counseling provided by the research team was also likely to have had an impact on participants' decision to choose a LARC method.

The study had a nonrandomized design, which impacts the ability to eliminate potential confounders associated with contraceptive choice and compliance.

Other Relevant Studies and Information:

- A state-wide initiative in Colorado (Colorado Family Planning Initiative) had similar findings as the CHOICE study. LARC were shown to be more effective than pills/patch/ring in reducing birth and abortion rates, particularly in adolescents and young women.[3]
- In both the CHOICE study and the Colorado Family Planning Initiative, more women chose LARC when available at no cost. The increase uptake in LARC was associated with a decrease in abortion rate and teen birth rate.[3,4]
- The American College of Obstetricians and Gynecologists, The American Academy of Pediatrics, the Centers of Disease Control and Prevention, and the Society of Family Planning have all endorsed LARC as safe for use in adolescents as in adults.[5–8]

Summary and Implications: The CHOICE study demonstrated that LARC are a highly effective form of birth control, leading to fewer unintended pregnancies compared to contraceptive pills, patch, or ring methods. Importantly, among adolescents, LARC are as effective in this cohort as in older women, but non-LARC methods (pills, patch, or contraceptive rings) are more likely to lead to unintended pregnancy. This study supports clinical guidelines supporting LARC use as first line for contraception among women of all age groups.

CLINICAL CASE

Case History
A 19-year-old G0P0 presents to your office and wants the most effective method of contraception. Her sister has a levonorgestrel intrauterine device and she is interested in one. She was told by another gynecologist that she could not have an IUD as she is too young and has never been pregnant. The patient wants your recommendations.

Suggested Answer
IUDs are safe for adolescents, and their use in this population is endorsed by all major professional organizations. In the adolescent population, LARC were demonstrated to be more effective for preventing pregnancy compared to pills/patch/ring. The patient should be counseled on reversible contraception including the benefits of LARC. Data have consistently shown that LARC are safe and effective reversible methods of contraception

in women of all ages. This patient should be able to obtain an IUD if that is her desired method.

Best practice would suggest, too, that lowering the financial barriers to LARC will increase uptake and that the majority of women will continue this method and be satisfied with it compared to shorter-acting methods.

References

1. Winner B, et al. Effectiveness of long-acting reversible contraception. *N Engl J Med.* 2012;366:1998–2007.
2. Secura GM, et al. The Contraceptive CHOICE Project: reducing barriers to long-acting reversible contraception. *Am J Obstet Gynecol.* 2010;203(2):115 e1–7.
3. Ricketts S, Klingler G, Schwalberg, R. Game change in Colorado: widespread use of long-acting reversible contraceptives and rapid decline in births among young, low-income women. *Perspect Sex Reprod Health.* 2014;46(3):125–132.
4. Secura GM, et al. Provision of no-cost, long-acting contraception and teenage pregnancy. *N Engl J Med.* 2014;371:1316–1323.
5. ACOG Committee Opinion No. 735: adolescents and long-acting reversible contraception: implants and intrauterine devices. *Obstet Gynecol.* 2018;131(5):e130–e139.
6. Committee on Practice Bulletins-Gynecology, Practice Bulletin No. 186: long-acting reversible contraception: implants and intrauterine devices. *Obstet Gynecol.* 2017;130(5):e251–e269.
7. Ott MA, Sucato GS, Committee on Adolescene. Contraception for adolescents. *Pediatrics.* 2014;134(4):e1257–e1281.
8. Curtis KM, et al. U.S. medical eligibility criteria for contraceptive use, 2016. *MMWR Recomm Rep.* 2016;65(3):1–103.
9. Lohr PA, Lyus R, Prager, S. Use of intrauterine devices in nulliparous women. *Contraception.* 2017;95(6):529–537.
10. Peipert JF, et al. Continuation and satisfaction of reversible contraception. *Obstet Gynecol.* 2011;117(5):1105–1113.
11. O'Neil-Callahan M., et al. Twenty-four-month continuation of reversible contraception. *Obstet Gynecol.* 2013;122(5):1083–1091.
12. Diedrich JT, et al. Three-year continuation of reversible contraception. *Am J Obstet Gynecol,* 2015;213(5):662 e1–8.

29

Long-Acting Reversible Contraception (LARC) and Teen Pregnancy

The Contraceptive CHOICE Project

JACLYN GRENTZER

"Teenage girls and women who were provided contraception at no cost and educated about reversible contraception and the benefits of LARC methods had rates of pregnancy, birth, and abortion that were much lower than the national rates for sexually experienced teens."

—GM SECURA ET AL.[1]

Research Question: Does removal of economic, educational, and logistical barriers to use of LARC, including intrauterine devices (IUDs) and the contraceptive implant, reduce pregnancy, birth, and abortion rates among sexually active teens?

Funding: Grants from the Susan Thompson Buffett Foundation, the Eunice Kennedy Shriver National Institute of Child Health and Human Development, and the National Center for Advancing Translational Sciences

Study Years: 2007–2011

Publication Year: 2014

Study Location: St. Louis, Missouri

Who Was Studied: English- or Spanish-speaking women 15 to 19 years of age who were sexually active or planning to become sexually active in the next 6 months, desired pregnancy prevention for at least 1 year, and were willing to start or switch to a new contraceptive method

Who Was Excluded: Those who had undergone hysterectomy or permanent sterilization

How Many Patients: 1,404

Study Overview: See Figure 28.1

Study Intervention: CHOICE participants received standardized contraceptive counseling and were given their choice of reversible contraceptive method at no cost for the duration of the study period. Same-day start for all contraceptive methods, including LARC, was provided if there were no medical contraindications.

Follow-Up: Telephone interviews at 3 and 6 months and every 6 months thereafter for 2 to 3 years

Endpoints: Primary outcomes: Rates of pregnancy, live birth, and induced abortion per 1,000 women. These were reported as "teen years" by calculating the total amount of time that each participant was in the study and not pregnant. Secondary outcomes involved further analysis of these same rates according to age and race.

RESULTS

- 71.5% of teen girls chose LARC when barriers to contraceptive access were removed.
- In the CHOICE cohort rates of pregnancy, live birth, and induced abortion rates were lower than the US teen population rates. (See Table 29.1.)
- LARC (levonorgestrel IUD, copper IUD, and etonorgestrel contraceptive implant) and depo provera had the lowest failure rates at 5.1, 0, 0, and 5.2 failures per 1000 teen years, respectively.
- Oral contraceptive pills, contraceptive ring and patch had higher failure rates of the contraceptive options evaluated at 56.8, 51.8, and 60.8 failures per 1000 teen years, respectively.

Criticisms and Limitations: One limitation of this study is that information about pregnancy and pregnancy outcomes was self-reported both in the study cohort and the US population data on teen pregnancies. This could have underestimated the rates of pregnancy. Furthermore, generalizability of these data are uncertain since study participants received standardized contraceptive counseling which may or not be provided in all contraceptive provision settings. In addition, members of the study cohort were contacted on a regular basis, which could have affected adherence to their contraceptive method. Additionally, teens in the study required parental consent to participate. Teens who feel comfortable obtaining parental consent could represent a group that are at lower risk for pregnancy or contraceptive non-use at baseline.

Other Relevant Studies and Information:

Table 29.1. REPRODUCTIVE OUTCOMES

Outcome	CHOICE Cohort	US Population, Sexually Experienced Teens	US Population, All Teens
Pregnancy	34.0	158.5	57.4
Birth	19.4	94.0	34.4
Abortion	9.7	41.5	14.7

Outcome is presented as number per 1000 teens.

- In 2014, only 10% of teens aged 15 to 19 reported using a LARC method.[2]
- Teen continuation rates at 12 months of contraceptive use are higher for LARC (81%) than for non-LARC (44%).[3]
- Youth-friendly clinic practices increase LARC uptake among teens. These practices include evening clinic hours, walk-in availability, practicing evidence-based care with initiation of hormonal contraception without a pelvic exam (except for an IUD insertion), providing contraceptive education by peer educators, staff training on how to better communicate with and meet the needs of teens, and protocols for ensuring confidentiality and building trust.[4]
- Both the American Academy of Pediatrics (AAP) and the American College of Obstetrians and Gynecologists (ACOG) recommend LARC like IUDs and contraceptive implants as the first-line contraceptives for teens and adolescents.[5,6]

- The ACOG considers same-day insertion to be one of the top 4 best practices for LARC insertion.[7]

Summary and Implications: When teens receive standardized contraceptive counseling, and barriers to accessing all methods of contraception are removed, they are more likely to (a) choose highly effective LARC like IUDs and the contraceptive implant and (b) have lower pregnancy, live birth, and induced abortion rates as compared to national rates for sexually experienced US teens.

CLINICAL CASE: LONG-ACTING REVERSIBLE CONTRACEPTION (LARC) AND TEEN PREGNANCY

Case History

A 15-year-old G1P0010 with no medical comorbidities presents to your office for contraceptive counseling. She has a history of 1 prior induced abortion and is currently using condoms alone for contraception. She tells you that she wants a birth control method that is very effective and easy to use. Based on the Contraceptive CHOICE Project data for teen pregnancy, how would you counsel this patient?

Suggested Answer

The Contraceptive CHOICE Project data for teen pregnancy showed that providing standardized contraceptive counseling, as well as providing all methods of reversible contraception at no cost, results in higher uptake of LARC and subsequently decreased rates of teen pregnancy, live birth, and induced abortion.

Based on this data, as well as recommendations from both the American Academy of Pediatrics and the American College of Obstetricians and Gynecologists, this patient should be offered all methods of contraception for which she is eligible, with emphasis placed on LARC (IUDs and the contraceptive implant). If the patient desires LARC, then insertion should occur on the same day as the request as long as there are no medical contraindications.

References

1. Secura GM, Madden T, McNicholas C, Mullersman J, Buckel CM, Zhao Q, Peipert JF. Provision of no-cost, long-acting contraception and teenage pregnancy. *N Engl J Med.* 2014 Oct 2;371(14):1316–1323.

2. Kavanaugh ML, Jerman J. Contraceptive method use in the United States: trends and characteristics between 2008, 2012 and 2014. *Contraception*. 2018 Jan;97(1):14–21.

3. Rosenstock JR, Peipert JF, Madden T, Zhao Q, Secura GM. Continuation of reversible contraception in teenagers and young women. *Obstet Gynecol*. 2012 Dec;120(6):1298–1305.

4. Kavanaugh ML, Jerman J, Ethier K, Moskosky S. Meeting the contraceptive needs of teens and young adults: youth-friendly and long-acting reversible contraceptive services in U.S. family planning facilities. *J Adolesc Health*. 2013 Mar;52(3):284–292.

5. Committee on Adolescence. Contraception for adolescents. *Pediatrics*. 2014 Oct;134(4):e1244–e1256.

6. Committee on Adolescent Health Care. Committee Opinion No. 710: counseling adolescents about contraception. *Obstet Gynecol*. 2017 Aug;130(2):e74–e80.

7. Committee on Gynecologic Practice Long-Acting Reversible Contraception Working Group. Committee Opinion No. 642: increasing access to contraceptive implants and intrauterine devices to reduce unintended pregnancy. *Obstet Gynecol*. 2015 Oct;126(4):e44–e48.

30

Effect of Screening Mammography on Breast Cancer Detection and Mortality

MYRLENE JEUDY, MONIQUE SWAIN, AND MARK PEARLMAN

"Our analysis suggests that whatever the mortality benefit, breast-cancer screening involved a substantial harm of excess detection of additional early-stage cancers that was not matched by a reduction in late-stage cancers."

—A BLEYER AND B WELCH[1]

Research Question: Is mammography an effective screening tool that increases the detection of early-stage breast cancer, thus decreasing the incidence of late-stage breast cancer and breast cancer mortality?

Funding: Not reported

Study Years: 1976–2008

Year Study Published: 2012

Study Location: United States

Who Was Studied: The study model examined trends among women 40 years or older in the United States who underwent for screening mammography, using data from the National Health Interview Survey (NHIS), the Surveillance, Epidemiology and End Results (SEER) database, and census data. NHIS provides estimates of self-reported health measures, including utilization, in a nationally representative sample of individuals. SEER reports incidence and survival rates from cancer registries. The authors utilized the SEER 9 database, which includes reports of cancer incidence and survival data from 9 areas (5 states and four metropolitan cities) that represent 10% of the US population.

Who Was Excluded: Lobular carcinoma in situ was excluded from the model.

Study Intervention: Trend data was used to model utilization of screening mammography and incidence rates of breast cancer in women 40 years or older. The authors calculated a baseline rate (1976–1978) of stage-specific breast cancer incidence prior to implementation of universal screening recommendations and then estimated incidence of breast cancer from 2006 to 2008. These estimates took into account a calculation of the excess (or deficit) of the number of cancer cases detected during each subsequent year and also took into account the impact of hormone replacement therapy on an increased risk of breast cancer diagnosis. The authors provided a range of assumptions in the annual percent change (APC) of breast cancer incidence to account for inaccuracies in their estimates.

Follow-Up: Not applicable

Endpoints: Absolute reduction of late-stage breast cancer

RESULTS

- The study's model suggested that in the 30 years following the introduction of screening mammography, detection of early-stage breast cancer had increased from 112 to 234 cases (a 122-case increase) per 100,000 women, while the detection of late-stage breast cancer had fallen from 102 to 94 cases (an 8-case decrease) per 100,000 women. This represented an excess detection of 114 cases of early breast cancer that would not have progressed to late-stage breast cancer. See Table 30.1.
- The increase in detection of early-stage breast cancer was driven by an 8-fold increase in the detection of Ducal Carcinoma In Situ (DCIS) and a 68.6% increase in the detection of localized disease. The decrease in the detection of late-stage breast cancer was driven by the increased detection of regional disease.
- When extrapolated to the population of women as a whole, the authors estimated that based on a stable incidence of cancer, 1.3 million women over the 30-year period would have been impacted by excess detection of early breast cancer that would not progress to late-stage cancer.

Table 30.1. ESTIMATES OF THE EXCESS DETECTION (OVERDIAGNOSIS) OF BREAST
CANCER ASSOCIATED WITH 3 DECADES OF MAMMOGRAPHY SCREENING

	Surplus in Diagnosis of Early-Stage Breast Cancer	Reduction of Late-Stage Diagnosis	Excess Detection
Base cases (based on SEER data)	1,518,000	67,000	1,518,000
Expected detection based on 0.25% APC	1,507,000	138,000	1,369,000
Expected detection based on 0.50% APC	1,426,000	213,000	1,213,000
Expected detection based on 0.50% APC and highest baseline incidence of late-stage disease observed	1,426,000	410,000	1,016,000

Abbreviations: SEER, Surveillance, Epidemiology and End Results; APC, annual
percent change.

- Assumptions regarding increases in incidence of breast cancer were incorporated to include an increase in breast cancer incidence and an increase in the initial baseline incidence of late-stage disease to reflect the highest observed incidence in the 30-year data reported by SEER. At the "very extreme" of these assumptions (representing an 0.5% APC in breast cancer per year and a baseline incidence of late-stage cancer of 113 cases per 100,000 women), the authors extrapolated a 410,000 reduction in the number of women diagnosed with late-stage disease and 1,016,000 cases of excess detection of early-stage cancer.
- The base case estimate assumes the incidence of breast cancer is constant, excluding transient cases attributable to hormone replacement therapy). A 0.25% APC is equivalent to the increased incidence observed among women younger than 40 who do not routinely receive screening mammogram.

Criticisms and Limitations: The study and its conclusions proved controversial, illustrating a particular tension in the development of screening guidelines in breast cancer, which attempt to balance real reductions in the rate of morbidity and mortality of breast cancer with the increase in early diagnosis that may lead to excess diagnostic procedures, patient worry, and health care burden.

The most prominent criticism of this study is that the model assumptions regarding the APC in breast cancer incidence may be too conservative, even at the most "extreme" assumption of 0.50%, as the estimate appears to be lower than other reported long-range APC estimates in both the United States and Europe.[2-6] A 40-year database of APC in Connecticut demonstrated a 1.2% APC. Utilizing this APC, the impact on late-stage cancer decrease would be 37% (as opposed to 8% using the 0.25% APC) and a nearly reciprocal 48% increase in early stage disease (not 69%).

The SEER database further does not provide specific information regarding the mammogram utilization; it may not be fully accurate to assume that all women in the early time frame (1976–1978) did not undergo mammographic diagnosis, nor that all women in the later time frame (2006–2008) did; the CDC reported that 81.1% of women ages 50 to 74 reported receiving an up-to-date mammogram in 2008.[7]

Subsequent studies have, with more generous assumptions regarding the annual percentage of change of breast cancer, suggested a real reduction in mortality at higher APC, as do other various trials and observational studies, despite flaws.

Other Relevant Studies and Information: A re-analysis of the SEER data broadened initial assumptions regarding APC and found that when APC was assumed to be 1% or greater, the rate of invasive cancers decreased.[8] Several other randomized control trials and population studies have also demonstrated a reduction in mortality of breast cancer.[8]

The Cochrane review conducted a meta-analysis of 8 trials that compared mammography screening and found a relative risk reduction of 0.81 for breast cancer mortality, although the 3 trials with adequate randomized found that mammography did not impact cancer mortality or all-cause mortality, and the total numbers of lumpectomies and mastectomies were significantly larger in the screened groups.[9]

National guidelines regarding breast cancer screening continue to vary. The American College of Obstetricians and Gynecologists recommends offering screening beginning at age 40 and continuing annually as long as the woman is in good health; this is representative of most other major US guidelines. The US Preventive Task Force represents the least conservative screening guidelines, recommending screening every 2 years starting at age 50, stopping at age 74.[10,11]

Summary and Implications: This observational study modeled SEER data to demonstrate a probable decrease in advanced breast cancer with an increase in the detection of early breast cancer, assuming a range of estimated annual percentage change of breast cancer. The results of this study suggested overdiagnosis with minimal impact on late-stage breast cancer reduction.

CLINICAL CASE

Case History
A 50-year-old healthy female presents for her annual gynecological annual. She has no personal or family history of breast cancer. She has never had a breast biopsy. She is not on any medications. She would like to discuss the risk and benefits of mammography for breast cancer screening.

How should this woman be counseled regarding breast cancer screening?

Suggested Answer
Risk has been assessed for this patient, and she appears to be of average risk (without a family history of breast or ovarian cancer, or cancer syndromes, BRCA-1 or BRCA-2, a history of earlier chest radiation, or a history of high-risk breast biopsy results).

The patient is 50 and is at the age at which all national guidelines recommend mammogram should been initiated with the expected benefit of breast cancer mortality improvement based on multiple prospective, randomized controlled trials.[11] As with any screening test, a full, nuanced conversation regarding the utility of screening should include a discussion that any screening test is liable to both false negatives (leading to late diagnosis of existing pathology) and false positives (leading to anxiety and the potential or additional procedures).

References

1. Bleyer A, Welch HG. Effect of three decades of screening mammography on breast-cancer incidence. *N Engl J Med.* 2012;367(21):1998–2005. doi:10.1056/NEJMoa1206809
2. Bray F, McCarron P, Parkin DM. The changing global patterns of female breast cancer incidence and mortality. *Breast Cancer Res.* 2004. doi:10.1186/bcr932
3. Holford TR, Cronin KA, Mariotto AB, Feuer EJ. Changing patterns in breast cancer incidence trends. *J Natl Cancer Inst Monogr.* 2006. doi:10.1093/jncimonographs/lgj016
4. Prior P. Reliability of underlying incidence rates for estimating the effect and efficiency of screening for breast cancer. *J Med Screen.* 1996. doi:10.1177/096914139600300303

5. Stevens RG, Moolgavkar SH, Lee JAH. Temporal trends in breast cancer. *Am J Epidemiol.* 1982. doi:10.1093/oxfordjournals.aje.a113358

6. Joensuu H, Toikkanen S. Comparison of breast carcinomas diagnosed in the 1980s with those diagnosed in the 1940s to 1960s. *Br Med J.* 1991. doi:10.1109/31.1842

7. Centers for Disease Control and Prevention. Vital signs: breast cancer screening among women aged 50–74 years—United States, 2008. *MMWR Morb Mortal Wkly Rep.* 2010; 59(26):813–816.

8. Helvie MA, Chang JT, Hendrick RE, Banerjee M. Reduction in late-stage breast cancer incidence in the mammography era: implications for overdiagnosis of invasive cancer. *Cancer.* 2014. doi:10.1002/cncr.28784

9. Gøtzsche PC, Jørgensen K. Screening for breast cancer with mammography. *Cochrane Database Sys Rev.* 2013;6:CD001877. doi:10.1002/14651858.CD001877.pub5

10. Garfinkel L, Boring CC, Heath CW. Changing trends: an overview of breast cancer incidence and mortality. *Cancer.* 1994. doi:10.1002/cncr.2820741304

11. Tabár L, Dean PB, Chen THH, et al. The incidence of fatal breast cancer measures the increased effectiveness of therapy in women participating in mammography screening. *Cancer.* 2018. doi:10.1002/cncr.31840

12. Oeffinger KC, Fontham ET, Etzioni R, Herzig A, Michaelson JS, Shih YC, et al. Breast cancer screening for women at average risk: 2015 guideline update from the American Cancer Society. *JAMA.* 2015;314(15):1599–1614.

Human Papillomavirus Infection of the Cervix

Relative Risk Association of 15 Common Anogenital Types

JACQUELINE M. MILLS AND ELIZABETH A. STIER

"HPV 6/11, 42, 43 and 44 were detected most frequently in low-grade lesions, in keeping with their low-risk status. Types 31,33,35,51,52 and 58 were most common in intraepithelial than invasive lesions, thus justifying the term intermediate risk. Conversely, HPVs 16,18,45 and 56 were most prominently associated with invasive cancer."

—AT LORINCZ ET AL.[1]

Research Question: Is there a correlation between detected cervical human papillomavirus (HPV) genotypes and cervical pathology?

Funding: Not reported

Study Years: 1982–1989

Year Study Published: 1992

Study Location: 8 centers in the United States and South America

Who Was Studied: This study included stored cervical specimens (swabs or biopsies) from women participating in cervical HPV studies conducted in the 1980s

Who Was Excluded: Not stated

How Many Patients: 2,627

Study Overview: See Figure 31.1

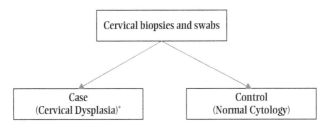

Figure 31.1. Study overview
*Including atypical, low-grade dysplasia, high-grade dysplasia, and cancer.

Study Intervention: Previously collected cervical biopsies and swabs were categorized by grade of cervical disease—normal cervical cytology and normal cervigram (controls), atypia, low-grade, high-grade, or cancer. Each of the specimens was then reanalyzed for detection of HPV genotype(s) (including HPVs 31, 33, 35, 42, 43, 44, 45, 51, 52, 56, and 58 in addition to the prior testing for HPVs 6, 11, 16, and 18). Analyses were then done to assess patterns of association between grade of cervical disease and the different HPV genotypes.

Follow-Up: None

Endpoints: Stratifying HPV genotyping results by cytologic/histologic diagnosis

---

RESULTS

- HPV DNA was detected in 79.3% of cases with cancer, High-Grade Squamous Intraepithelial Lesion, or Low-Grade Squamous Intraepithelial Lesion and was detected in 23.7% of cases with atypia of uncertain significance. HPV DNA was found in only 6.4% of controls with negative cytology and/or colposcopy. See Table 31.1.
- Strains of HPV were risk-stratified into low-risk, intermediate-risk and high-risk groups based on their prevalence in premalignant and malignant cervical lesions.

Table 31.1. SUMMARY OF KEY FINDINGS

HPV Genotype

		6/11, 42, 43, 44 (low–risk)	31, 33, 35, 51, 52 (intermediate risk)	18, 45, 56 (high–risk)	16 (high–risk)
	RR (95% CI)	6.1 (3.1–12.1)	2.6 (1.2–5.2)	6.6 (2.8– 15.7)	5.0 (2.5–9.9)
	% cases by Diagnosis (#)	4.8% (13/270)	3.7% (10/270)	3.0% (8/270)	4.4% (12/270)
LSIL	RR (95% CI)	52.6 (36.0–76.9)	21.6 (17.9–26.1)	32.7 (19.2–55.8)	36.9 (25.0–54.5)
	% cases by Diagnosis (#)	20.2% (76/377)	15.4% (58/377)	7.2% (27/377)	16.2% (61/377)
HSIL	RR (95% CI)	24.1 (13.4–43.4)	71.9 (51.0–101.6)	65.1 (50.2–84.5)	235.7 (198.5–279.5)
	% cases by Diagnosis (#)	4.2% (11/261)	23.4% (61/261)	6.5% (17/261)	47.1% (123/261)
Invasive Cancer	RR (95% CI)	0 (0–0)	31.1 (18.7–51.8)	296.1 (198.9–441.1)	260 (216.9–311.9)
	% cases by Diagnosis (#)	0% (0/153)	9.2% (14/153)	26.8% (41/153)	47.1% (72/153)

Abbreviations: CI, confidence interval; HPV, human papilloma virus; RR, Relative Risk; SIL, squamous intraepithelial lesions.

- Low-risk strains (6, 11, 42, 43, and 44) were present in 20.2% (76 of 377) of low-grade lesions and not detected in any of the 153 cancers.
- Intermediate-risk strains (31, 33, 35, 51, 52, and 58) were detected in 23.8% (62 of 261) of high-grade squamous intraepithelial lesions and 10.5% (16 of 153) of cancers.
- High-risk strains (18, 45, and 56) were found in 6.5% (17 of 261) of high-grade intraepithelial lesions and in 26.8% (41 of 153) of invasive carcinomas.
- HPV 16 was considered in its own high-risk category, as this strain alone was associated with 47.1% of high-grade intraepithelial lesions (123 of 261) and 47.1% of cancers (72 of 153).

Criticisms and Limitations: The primary limitation of this study is that it is a reanalysis of stored specimens from 8 different studies that were neither designed nor powered to determine the association of HPV genotype (with the current method of assessment) with grade of cervical neoplasia. It is notable that several other oncogenic HPV subtypes, (39, 59, 66, and 69) were not tested in this analysis. Additionally, because the DNA sequence of HPV 58 was not available until late in the analysis, only a subset of samples in the study were assessed for HPV 58.

Other Relevant Studies and Information:

- HPV has been demonstrated to be a cause of invasive cervical cancer worldwide.[2]
- A long-term prospective study of type-specific HPV infection and risk of cervical neoplasia among 20,000 women in the Portland Kaiser cohort study demonstrated that HPV prevalence has a strong association with high-grade cervical dysplasia and cervical cancer and that the risk of CIN-3 or cervical cancer was highest with HPV 16.[3]
- Screening strategies that incorporate cytology, HPV testing, and genotyping for HPV 16/18 appear to maximize sensitivity and minimize the number of unnecessary colposcopies.[4] The American College of Obstetricians and Gynecologists, the American Society for Colposcopy and Cervical Pathology, and the American Cancer Society support HPV co-testing as the preferred primary screening method, based on the strength of association between high-risk HPV and cervical dysplasia.

Summary and Implications: Lorincz et al. evaluated the clinicopathologic correlation with a broad subset of HPV genotypes with oncogenic potential. Their analyses found that (a) HPV infection is strongly correlated with cervical cancer risk, (b) detection of the cancer associated HPV genotypes may help to identify women at risk for cervical pre-cancer and cancer, and (c) a prophylactic HPV vaccine should include protection against the most strongly oncogenic HPV strains, such as HPV 16 and 18.

CLINICAL CASE

Case History

A 45-year-old woman with no history of abnormal pap tests (most recent test was normal from 3 years prior) presents to her primary provider's office for routine cervical cancer screening. The results of her screening (co-testing) included a normal cervical cytology and a positive HPV test (negative for HPV types 16 and 18). Her provider recommends she have another co-test in 1 year. The patient is upset that nothing is recommended for now and presents to you for a second opinion. Does the patient need a colposcopy now? Is it safe to wait a year?

Suggested Answer

Management of abnormal cervical cancer screening is based on the risk of CIN3+ for a given population. For a woman with normal cytology associated with HPV (non-16,18) the risk of CIN3+ is 2%[2] and the risk of cancer is close to 0. Therefore the recommendations are to repeat the co-testing in 1 year and if either is abnormal at that time, then the recommendation at that time is for referral for colposcopy. In comparison, a woman with a normal cervical cytology and a positive test for HPV 16,18 has a 9% risk of CIN3+[5] and would be recommended for colposcopy.

We would counsel the patient that she does not require colposcopy at this time because (a) the HPV may "clear" within the year, and it is only persistent HPV infections that are associated with cancer and (b) her current risk for CIN3 is negligible. We recommend she undergo co-testing in 1 year to assess for persistent HPV infection, allowing her to likely avoid the many costs associated with colposcopic evaluation.

References

1. Lorincz AT, Reid R, Jenson AB, Greenberg MD, Lancaster W, Kurman RJ. Human papillomavirus infection of the cervix: relative risk associations of 15 common anogenital types. *Obstet Gynecol.* 1992;79(3):328–337. http://www.ncbi.nlm.nih.gov/pubmed/1310805.
2. Walboomers JM, Jacobs MV, Manos MM, et al. Human papillomavirus is a necessary cause of invasive cervical cancer worldwide. *J Pathol.* 1999;189(1):12–19. doi:10.1002/(SICI)1096-9896(199909)189:1<12::AID-PATH431>3.0.CO;2-F.
3. Schiffman M, Glass AG, Wentzensen N, et al. A long-term prospective study of type-specific human papillomavirus infection and risk of cervical neoplasia among 20,000 women in the Portland Kaiser Cohort Study [published correction appears in Cancer Epidemiol Biomarkers Prev. 2012 Aug;21(8):1390–1]. *Cancer Epidemiol Biomarkers Prev.* 2011;20(7):1398–1409. doi:10.1158/1055-9965.EPI-11-0206
4. Cox JT, Castle PE, Behrens CM, et al. Comparison of cervical cancer screening strategies incorporating different combinations of cytology, HPV testing, and genotyping for HPV 16/18: results from the ATHENA HPV study. *Am J Obstet Gynecol.* 2013;208(3):184.e1–184.e11. doi:10.1016/j.ajog.2012.11.020
5. Wentzensen N, Clarke MA, Bremer R, et al. Clinical Evaluation of human papillomavirus screening with p16/Ki-67 dual stain triage in a large organized cervical cancer screening program. *JAMA Intern Med.* May 2019. doi:10.1001/jamaintern med.2019.0306

32

Transvaginal Ultrasound for Endometrial Assessment of Postmenopausal Bleeding

ALISON A. GARRETT AND SARAH E. TAYLOR

"The current findings indicate that with 4mm as a cutoff limit transvaginal ultrasonography of the endometrium in a woman with postmenopausal bleeding can exclude abnormality with reasonable certainty."
—B KARLSSON ET AL.[1]

Research Question: Can transvaginal ultrasonographic measurement of endometrial thickness be used to exclude endometrial abnormalities in women with postmenopausal bleeding?

Funding: Swedish Medical Research Foundation, Goteborg Medical Society, B&S Medical

Year Study Began: 1989

Year Study Published: 1995

Study Location: 9 hospitals in Sweden, Finland, Denmark, and Norway

Who Was Studied: This is a multicenter study consisting of women with postmenopausal bleeding who were admitted to participating hospitals for a curettage. A woman was considered postmenopausal if more than 1 year had elapsed since her last menstrual period. Of the 1168 women included in the study, 351 women were receiving hormonal replacement therapy (165 receiving estriol and 186 receiving systemic hormone replacement therapy with estrogen-progestin therapy).

Who Was Excluded: None

How Many Patients: 1,168

Study Overview: See Figure 32.1 for a summary of the study design.

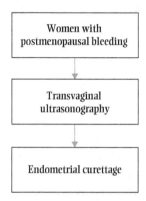

Figure 32.1. Study overview

Study Intervention: Eligible subjects underwent transvaginal ultrasonography followed by endometrial curettage. Transvaginal ultrasound was performed either on the same day or up to 3 days before curettage.

Follow-Up: None

Endpoints: The primary endpoint was the detection of an endometrial abnormality on histopathology.

RESULTS

- Histopathology of curettage specimens diagnosed 667 cases of atrophy, 77 cases of hormonal effect, 140 endometrial polyps, 114 endometrial cancers, and 112 cases of hyperplasia.
- The endometrial thickness was unable to be measured in 30 women (2.8%). For these women, curettage demonstrated one endometrial cancer, 1 hyperplasia without atypia, 1 stage IV cervical cancer, 5 polyps, 1 hematometra, 19 cases of atrophy, and 2 cases of hormonal effect.

- The probability of finding an endometrial abnormality was 3.6% for an endometrial thickness of ≤4mm (including 6 cases of endometrial hyperplasia and 6 endometrial polyps), 6.1% for an endometrial thickness ≤5mm, and 8.5% for an endometrial thickness ≤6mm. No endometrial cancers were detected at an endometrial thickness cutoff of 4mm. Two endometrial cancers were detected at a cutoff of 5mm.
- The sensitivity for detecting a histologically abnormal endometrium for an endometrial thickness ≤4mm was 96%, the specificity was 68%, and the negative predictive value was 97%.
- The authors of this paper report that by using a 4mm cutoff limit, the number of endometrial sampling procedures could have been reduced by 46%.

Table 32.1. HISTOLOGIC DIAGNOSIS OF CURETTAGE SPECIMENS AND CORRESPONDING ENDOMETRIAL THICKNESS

Diagnosis	Endometrial Thickness (mm)					Total
	≤4	5	6–10	11–20	>20	
Endometrial abnormality	14 (2.7%)	10 (11.4%)	112 (45.7%)	168 (80.0%)	71 (92.2%)	375 (33.0%)
Endometrial polyp	6	5	54	58	17	140
Hyperplasia	6	2	41	53	10	112
Endometrial Cancer	0	2	13	55	44	114
Cervical Cancer	2	1	4	2	0	9
Benign pathology [a]	504 (97.3%)	78 (88.6%)	133 (54.3%)	42 (20.0%)	6 (7.8%)	763 (67.0%)

[a]Includes atrophy, hormonal effect, and other.

Criticisms and Limitations: Accurate measurement of the endometrial lining is critical. Ultrasound technique and the use of experienced ultrasound examiners play an important role in assessing this measurement. Technical error, interexaminer variability, and availability of experienced sonographers may limit the value of these results in other locations.

This study was conducted in Denmark, Finland, Sweden, and Norway. Additionally, no patient demographic factors were recorded except for patient age. The generalizability of these results to other populations is not clear.

Other Relevant Studies and Information:

- Other studies evaluating the use of endometrial thickness to detect endometrial cancer have demonstrated similar sensitivities, specificities, and negative predictive values for varying endometrial thickness cutoffs. However, recommendations on what cutoff value to use in clinical practice vary slightly, with several studies recommending using ≤3mm as a cutoff versus ≤4mm.[2-5]

- The American College of Obstetricians and Gynecologists (ACOG) Committee on Gynecologic Practice recommends that postmenopausal bleeding requires evaluation either with transvaginal ultrasonography or endometrial sampling with endometrial biopsy or curettage to exclude or diagnose endometrial cancer. The guidelines recommend that if the endometrial thickness is ≤4mm on transvaginal ultrasonography, no further workup is indicated given the high negative predictive value for endometrial cancer in this setting. For women with recurrent bleeding or persistent bleeding, or for women on tamoxifen with postmenopausal bleeding, endometrial sampling is recommended regardless of the endometrial thickness is on ultrasound.[5]

Summary and Implications: This study demonstrated that measurement of endometrial thickness by transvaginal ultrasonography is a reasonable initial strategy for the evaluation of postmenopausal bleeding. The negative predictive value for any endometrial abnormality is 97% with an endometrial thickness of ≤4mm, and no cases of endometrial cancer were detected in patients with an endometrial thickness ≤4mm. This suggests that for women with an episode of postmenopausal bleeding and an endometrial thickness ≤4mm, expectant management rather than endometrial biopsy is a reasonable option.

CLINICAL CASE: TRANSVAGINAL ULTRASONOGRAPHY FOR ENDOMETRIAL ASSESSMENT

Case History

A 64-year-old postmenopausal female with no significant past medical history presents with 2 episodes of vaginal spotting over the last month. She has no other symptoms. Transvaginal ultrasound is performed and reveals an endometrial thickness of 5mm and no other abnormalities. Based on the results of the Karlsson et al. study, what is the next best step in management?

Suggested Answer

Karlsson et al. demonstrated a high negative predictive value for endometrial abnormalities for women with postmenopausal bleeding and an endometrial thickness ≤4mm on transvaginal ultrasonography. For women with postmenopausal bleeding and an endometrial thickness >4mm, the negative predictive value for endometrial abnormalities decreases. Additionally, in this study there were 2 cases of endometrial cancer detected in women with an endometrial thickness of 5mm. Thus, the next most appropriate step in management is to perform endometrial sampling given the small risk of missing a diagnosis of endometrial cancer. Additionally, evaluating for other causes of vaginal bleeding in the postmenopausal patient is necessary, including ensuring up-to-date cervical cancer screening as well as assessing for vaginal atrophy. It is also important to note that for women with recurrent or persistent postmenopausal bleeding, even in the setting of an endometrial thickness ≤4mm on transvaginal ultrasonography, further workup with endometrial sampling is recommended.

References

1. Karlsson B, Granberg S, Wikland M, et al. Transvaginal ultrasonography of the endometrium in women with postmenopausal bleeding—a Nordic multicenter study. *Am J Obstet Gynecol.* 1995;172(5):1488–1494.
2. Ferrazzi E, Torri V, Trio D, Zannoni E, Filiberto S, Dordoni D. Sonographic endometrial thickness: a useful test to predict atrophy in patients with postmenopausal bleeding. An Italian multicenter study. *Ultrasound Obstet Gynecol.* 1996;7(5):315–321.
3. Timmermans A, Opmeer BC, Khan KS, et al. Endometrial thickness measurement for detecting endometrial cancer in women with postmenopausal bleeding: a systematic review and meta-analysis. *Obstet Gynecol.* 2010;116(1):160–167.
4. Wong ASW, Lao TTH, Cheung CW, et al. Reappraisal of endometrial thickness for the detection of endometrial cancer in postmenopausal bleeding: a retrospective cohort study. *BJOG.* 2016;123(3):439–446.
5. ACOG Committee Opinion No. 440: the role of transvaginal ultrasonography in evaluating the endometrium of women with postmenopausal bleeding. *Obset Gynecol.* 2018;131:e124–e129.

33

The Accuracy of Endometrial Sampling in the Diagnosis of Patients With Endometrial Carcinoma and Hyperplasia

A Meta-Analysis

CHELSEA CHANDLER AND ALEXANDER OLAWAIYE

"The Pipelle device is superior to other techniques in endometrial sampling, especially in postmenopausal women, for the detection of endometrial carcinoma and atypical hyperplasia."

—DIJKHUIZEN ET AL.[1]

Research Question: How accurate is endometrial sampling in the diagnosis of patients with endometrial carcinoma and atypical hyperplasia?

Funding: None reported

Years of Study: January 1966 to May 1999

Year Study Published: 2000

Study Location: This is a meta-analysis by authors based in the Netherlands that includes studies performed worldwide.

Who Was Studied: All previously published studies comparing the results of endometrial sampling with pathologic findings at the time of dilation and curettage (D&C), hysteroscopy, or hysterectomy.

Who Was Excluded: Studies on endometrial sampling that did not directly compare sampling results with reference pathologic findings.

How Many Patients: 7,814

Study Overview: See Figure 33.1

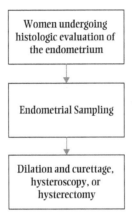

Figure 33.1. Study overview

This study was a meta-analysis of 39 studies published between January 1966 through May 1999 that compared the results of endometrial sampling with pathologic findings at the time of D&C, hysteroscopy, or hysterectomy. For each study, the number of patients in whom endometrial carcinoma and atypical hyperplasia were correctly identified at time of endometrial sampling was reported, along with the number of women in whom sampling failed. The authors also abstracted, if available, the menopausal status of study participants, symptomatic or asymptomatic nature, type of sampling (direct biopsy of the endometrium or indirect sampling through assessment of endometrial cells alone), pathologic reference strategy, as well as independence of assessment.

Endpoints: Primary endpoint: Sensitivity of endometrial sampling methods stratified by ability to detect endometrial carcinoma and atypical hyperplasia. Secondary endpoint: Percentage of patients where sampling did not provide a diagnosis.

RESULTS

- The sample-size weighted sensitivity of endometrial sampling with regards to detection of endometrial carcinoma is higher in postmenopausal women than premenopausal women (95% in studies including only postmenopausal women vs. 75% in all other studies including both pre- and postmenopausal women).
- The pipelle was the best device for detection of both atypical hyperplasia and endometrial carcinoma. In postmenopausal women the sensitivity for endometrial carcinoma with the pipelle is 99.6% and in studies including premenopausal women, 91%. With the pipelle, the sensitivity for atypical hyperplasia is 81% (the authors were not able to calculate sensitivity for pre- and postmenopausal women separately).

Table 33.1. SUMMARY OF STUDY'S KEY FINDINGS

Menopausal Status	Sensitivity of Pipelle (%)	Specificity of Pipelle (%)
Postmenopausal	99.6	95
Premenopausal	91	100

- Sensitivity of the Vabra device was 97.1% in postmenopausal women; in analyses that included premenopausal women the sensitivity was 80%. Endometrial lavage, an indirect method of detection, has a 57% sensitivity for detection of endometrial cancer.
- Failure of these methods to obtain endometrial sample sufficient for diagnosis was 10.4% with the pipelle, and 9.5% with other methods of endometrial sampling.

Criticisms and Limitations: The authors included a broad selection of studies investigating the accuracy of direct and indirect endometrial sampling in diagnosing endometrial carcinoma and atypical hyperplasia; however, there exists the potential for publication bias which would likely lead to an overestimation of the accuracy of pipelle sampling.

An additional limitation is that the studies included in this meta-analysis were heterogenous in their design and in endometrial sampling methods; only 15 of the included studies used the pipelle for sampling. The majority of studies reported on results using sampling methods, such as the Vabra aspirator or endometrial lavage, which are not in common use today.

The methods of pathology confirmation did differ among the included studies. Over half of included studies used dilation and curettage (generally considered the gold standard) as the reference test; 27% of studies included hysterectomy results. D&C has a reported false negative rate as high as 10%,[2] which may also impact meta-analysis results.

Other Relevant Studies and Information:

- The American College of Obstetricians and Gynecologists recommends outpatient endometrial sampling as the method of choice for histologic evaluation of the endometrium.[3]
- Acceptable less invasive options for initial evaluation of postmenopausal bleeding may include the use of transvaginal ultrasound.[4,5]
- Further evaluation of the uterine cavity is indicated in postmenopausal women with persistent bleeding even if with an initial benign endometrial sampling with pipelle.[6,7] Should further evaluation be required, D&C with hysteroscopy is recommended for accuracy and diagnostic yield.[3]

Summary and Implications: This meta-analysis of the diagnostic accuracy of endometrial sampling in pre- and postmenopausal women found that the sensitivity and specificity of the pipelle in the diagnosis of carcinoma and atypical hyperplasia was higher than for other methods, making it the preferred approach to initial endometrial sampling, particularly in women with postmenopausal bleeding.

CLINICAL CASE: ACCURACY OF ENDOMETRIAL SAMPLING IN DIAGNOSIS OF CARCINOMA AND ATYPICAL HYPERPLASIA

Case History

A 64-year-old woman who underwent menopause at age 52 reports 2 weeks of menstrual-like bleeding. She denies any prior episodes of bleeding. She has had no recent unexpected weight loss and denies early satiety or other concerning symptoms. Her pelvic exam is notable for a 9-week sized uterus without discernable adnexal masses. Her recent pap smear was normal.

Based on the results of the reviewed meta-analysis and current clinical guidelines, how should this patient be advised regarding workup and evaluation?

Suggested Answer

The patient in this case illustrates a common gynecologic complaint in postmenopausal women. While endometrial curettage has been the historical gold standard in the workup of abnormal uterine bleeding, pipelle sampling offers an efficient, sensitive, low-cost option that can be performed in the office. It should be noted that evaluation of endometrial thickness on transvaginal ultrasound may also be considered as a reasonable first step in the workup of postmenopausal bleeding and the detection of endometrial cancer.

Persistent or recurrent postmenopausal bleeding after benign in office endometrial sampling should result in an evaluation of the uterine cavity with hysteroscopy and D&C. A biopsy indicating insufficient sample should also warrant a conversation regarding further workup as well.

References

1. Dijkhuizen FPHLJ, Mol BWJ, Brölmann HAM, Heintz APM. The accuracy of endometrial sampling in the diagnosis of patients with endometrial carcinoma and hyperplasia: a meta-analysis. *Cancer.* 2000;89:1765–1772.
2. Word B, Gravlee LC, Wideman GL. The fallacy of simple uterine curettage. *Obstet Gynecol.* 1958;12:642–647.
3. American College of Obstetricians and Gynecologists Practice Bulletin #149 Endometrial cancer. *Obstet Gynecol.* 2015 Apr;125(4):1006–1026.
4. Gupta JK, Chien PF, Voit D, Clark TJ, Khan KS. Ultra-sonographic endometrial thickness for diagnosing endometrial pathology in women with postmenopausal bleeding: a meta-analysis. *Acta Obstet Gynecol Scand.* 2002;81:799–816.
5. Jacobs I, et al. Sensitivity of transvaginal ultrasound screening for endometrial cancer in postmenopausal women: a case-control study within the UKCTOCS cohort. *Lancet Oncol.* 2011;12:48.
6. Wang J, Wieslander C, Hansen G, Cass I, Vasilev S, Holschneider CH. Thin endometrial echo complex on ultrasound does not reliably exclude type 2 endometrial cancers. *Gynecol Oncol.* 2006;101:120–125.
7. Adambekov S, et al. Patient and provider factors associated with endometrial pipelle sampling failure. *Gynecol Oncol.* 2017;144:324–328.

34

Elective Bilateral Oophorectomy Versus Ovarian Conservation at the Time of Benign Hysterectomy

JOHNNY YI AND MEGAN WASSON

"Bilateral oophorectomy is associated with increased mortality in women aged younger than 50 years who never used estrogen therapy and at no age is oophorectomy associated with increased survival."

—WH PARKER ET AL.[1]

Research Question: Does oophorectomy or ovarian conservation at the time of benign hysterectomy impact long-term mortality?

Funding: National Institutes of Health grant for Nurses' Health Study (NHS) data collection and cohort maintenance

Study Years: 1976–June 1, 2008

Year Study Published: 2013

Study Location: 11 most populous states in the United States

Who Was Studied: Female registered nurses ages 35 to 55 with a prior hysterectomy for benign disease

Who Was Excluded: Women with a history of gynecologic cancer, other cancers, coronary heart disease, stroke, or pulmonary embolus or women with unilateral or partial oophorectomy, oophorectomy performed before or after the hysterectomy, unknown age at time of hysterectomy, or unknown ovarian status at time of hysterectomy.

How Many Patients: 30,117

Study Overview: See Figure 34.1

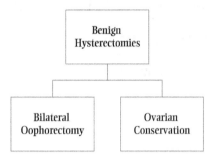

Figure 34.1. Study overview

This was a prospective cohort study assessing outcomes for participants who underwent bilateral oophorectomy versus ovarian conservation at the time of hysterectomy. Covariate data including BMI, family history of pertinent medical issues, medical history, gynecologic history, and social history were gathered. Multivariable adjusted hazard ratios for cause of death were applied to compare bilateral oophorectomy with ovarian conservation. Models were also fit with age at time of hysterectomy to identify the cutoff at which survival benefit of oophorectomy versus conservation might be conferred.

Follow-Up: Questionnaires administered every 2 years until death or 2008, constituting a total of 24 years of follow-up

Endpoints: Primary outcome: All-cause mortality. Secondary outcomes: Cause of death, including coronary heart disease, stroke, breast cancer, epithelial ovarian cancer, lung cancer, colorectal cancer, and total cancer

---

RESULTS

- Risk of overall mortality was significantly greater in patients who underwent bilateral oophorectomy at time of hysterectomy. Bilateral oophorectomy did not result in a lower risk of all-cause mortality in any age strata.

- Risk of death from ovarian cancer was lower among women receiving bilateral oophorectomy compared to ovarian conservation (0.33% vs. 0.024%), and risk of breast cancer was lower if the oophorectomy was performed before the age of 47.5 years.
- Risk of all-cause mortality was increased with concurrent oophorectomy if patients were low risk for cardiac disease. High-risk patients and patients who smoked did not incur additional mortality risk or risk of cardiovascular disease following oophorectomy in this analysis.
- Bilateral oophorectomy in women younger than 50 years was associated with a greater risk of all-cause mortality for women who had never used estrogen therapy.

Table 34.1. ALL-CAUSE MORTALITY INCIDENCE BY AGE

	Less Than 45 Years Old	45 to 54 Years Old	55 Years or Older	All Patients
Incidence of death with ovarian conservation at time of hysterectomy (per 100,000 person-years)	481	584	836	527
Incidence of death with oopherectomy at time of hysterectomy (per 100,000 person-years)	618	660	773	648
Age-adjusted HR (95% CI)[a]	1.18 (1.07–1.30)	1.17 (1.03–1.32)	1.10 (0.87–1.40)	1.10 (1.03–1.18)
Multivariate HR (95% CI)[a]	1.06 (0.95–1.18)	1.15 (1.01–1.32)	1.14 (0.85–1.52)	1.12 (1.03–1.21)

[a]Ovarian conservation is the reference group.
Abbreviations: HR, hazard ratio; CI, confidence interval.

Criticisms and Limitations: The primary limitation of this analysis is that it was not a randomized trial and as a result patients who received bilateral oophorectomy may have been different than those not receiving the procedure. As a result, confounding factors may have influenced the findings.

Subanalyses were likely underpowered to detect differences in mortality rates for women who have a family history of cancer or between women with high cardiac risk factors.

The NHS comprises a largely White, educated population, and the findings may not be generalizable to other populations.

Other Relevant Studies and Information:

- The American College of Obstetricians and Gynecologists recommends an informed discussion between patients and their surgeon regarding the risks and benefits of ovarian conservation. The benefits to ovarian conservation decrease after menopause with minimal benefit for ovarian conservation after age 65.[2]
- Other high-quality observations studies have similarly found that bilateral oophorectomy does not improve all-cause mortality and is associated with greater mortality particularly in younger, premenopausal women.[3–5]
- Other large studies have found other benefits for ovarian conservation compared with elective oophorectomy including lower rates of osteoporosis,[6] dementia and cognitive decline,[7] depression,[8] and glaucoma.[9]
- Current evidence suggests some protective effect from hormone replacement therapy following bilateral oophorectomy[3,4,10] this can be offered particularly for women who have bilateral oophorectomy prior to the age of 50.

Summary and Implications: This study found that women undergoing a bilateral oophorectomy at the time of a hysterectomy for benign gynecological conditions had increased mortality versus women who did not simultaneously receive an oophorectomy. Based on this and other studies, elective oophorectomy is not recommended for women younger than 50 or before menopause who are not at elevated risk for ovarian cancer or who do not have other compelling reasons for removal of the ovaries. The decision to offer an elective oophorectomy at the time of benign hysterectomy requires careful counseling regarding associated risks and should be individualized to take into account a patient's age, medical comorbidities, and any family history of breast or ovarian cancer.

CLINICAL CASE: COUNSELING A PATIENT REGARDING OVARIAN CONSERVATION VERSUS OOPHORECTOMY DURING BENIGN HYSTERECTOMY

Case History

A 48-year-old peri-menopausal woman with abnormal uterine bleeding due to adenomyosis is scheduled for a vaginal hysterectomy. She denies a personal history of cancer and does not have a family history of breast or ovarian cancer. She had a recent Pap smear and endometrial biopsy which were both normal. The patient has a friend who was recently diagnosed with Stage IIIC ovarian cancer and is wondering if she should have her ovaries removed to reduce her personal risk. During preoperative counseling, what will you counsel this patient regarding elective oophorectomy at the time of surgery?

Suggested Answer

Patients should be counseled that elective oophorectomy is associated with higher risk of death than ovarian conservation. This is particularly true for those below the age of 50 due to possible increased risk of cardiovascular disease and lung or colon cancer. There are other benefits to ovarian conservation including lower risk for depression, better cognitive outcomes, and potential decreased fractures as compared to patients who have their ovaries removed at the time of benign hysterectomy.

This patient does not have an apparent elevated risk for ovarian cancer. Therefore, she should be counseled that elective oophorectomy would decrease her risk of ovarian or primary peritoneal cancer. However, this benefit is outweighed by the increased risk of mortality from all other causes of death. In contrast, patients with known inherited cancer syndromes with predisposition to ovarian cancer should be counseled that oophorectomy may reduce their mortality. It is less clear whether patients with a family history of ovarian cancer, but without a known specific genetic cause, would benefit.

Absent other reasons to remove her ovaries, the clinician should recommend ovarian conservation in this patient. A careful presentation of the known and unknown risks for patients for bilateral oophorectomy should utilize a shared decision model to help the patient decide whether she should undergo elective oophorectomy.

References

1. Parker WH, Broder MS, Chang E, et al. Ovarian conservation at the time of hysterectomy and long-term health outcomes in the nurses' health study. *Obstet Gynecol.* 2009;113(5):1027–1037. doi:10.1097/AOG.0b013e3181a11c64.

2. ACOG Committee Opinion No. 774: Opportunistic Salpingectomy as a Strategy for Epithelial Ovarian Cancer Prevention. *Obstet Gynecol.* 2019;133(4):e279–e284. doi:10.1097/AOG.0000000000003164

3. Rocca WA, Grossardt BR, de Andrade M, Malkasian GD, Melton LJ. Survival patterns after oophorectomy in premenopausal women: a population-based cohort study. *Lancet Oncol.* 2006;7(10):821–828. doi:10.1016/S1470-2045(06)70869-5

4. Evans EC, Matteson KA, Orejuela FJ, et al. Salpingo-oophorectomy at the time of benign hysterectomy. *Obstet Gynecol.* 2016;128(3):476–485. doi:10.1097/AOG.0000000000001592.

5. Jacoby VL, Grady D, Wactawski-Wende J, et al. Oophorectomy vs ovarian conservation with hysterectomy. *Arch Intern Med.* 2011;171(8):760–768. doi:10.1001/archinternmed.2011.121.

6. Melton LJ, Khosla S, Malkasian GD, Achenbach SJ, Oberg AL, Riggs BL. Fracture risk after bilateral oophorectomy in elderly women. *J Bone Miner Res.* 2003;18(5):900–905. doi:10.1359/jbmr.2003.18.5.900

7. Rocca WA, Bower JH, Maraganore DM, et al. Increased risk of cognitive impairment or dementia in women who underwent oophorectomy before menopause. *Neurology.* 2007;69(11):1074–1083. doi:10.1212/01.wnl.0000276984.19542.e6

8. Chen X, Guo T, Li B. Influence of prophylactic oophorectomy on mood and sexual function in women of menopausal transition or postmenopausal period. *Arch Gynecol Obstet.* 2013;288(5):1101–1106. doi:10.1007/s00404-013-2865-1

9. Vajaranant TS, Grossardt BR, Maki PM, et al. Risk of glaucoma after early bilateral oophorectomy. *Menopause.* 2014;21(4):391–398. doi:10.1097/GME.0b013e31829fd081

10. Parker WH, Feskanich D, Broder MS, et al. Long-term mortality associated with oophorectomy compared with ovarian conservation in the nurses' health study. *Obstet Gynecol.* 2013;121(4):709–716. doi:10.1097/AOG.0b013e3182864350

35

Native-Tissue Anterior Colporrhaphy Versus Transvaginal Mesh for Anterior Pelvic Organ Prolapse

NICK ROCKEFELLER AND PETER JEPPSON

"As compared with anterior colporrhaphy, use of a standardized, trocar-guided mesh kit for cystocele repair resulted in higher short-term rates of successful treatment but also in higher rates of surgical complications and postoperative adverse events."

—D ALTMAN ET AL.[1]

Research Question: Should patients with anterior vaginal wall prolapse be managed with a traditional native tissue colporrhaphy or with transvaginal mesh?

Funding: Karolinska Institutet; Ethicon (medical device company)

Year Study Began: 2007

Year Study Published: 2011

Study Location: 53 hospitals throughout Sweden, Norway, Finland, and Denmark

Who Was Studied: Women with symptomatic primary or recurrent Stage 2 or higher anterior vaginal wall prolapse

Who Was Excluded: Women with prior pelvic organ cancer, current systemic glucocorticoid treatment, insulin-treated diabetes, need for concomitant surgery, or inability to complete study follow-up or provide informed consent.

How Many Patients: 389

Study Overview: See Figure 35.1

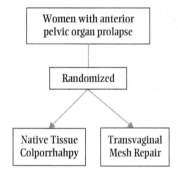

Figure 35.1. Study overview

Study Interventions: This randomized control trial assigned patients to traditional native-tissue anterior colporrhaphy or to a transvaginal trocar-guided mesh repair (Gynecare Prolift Anterior Pelvic Floor Repair System kit [Ethicon]).

Follow-Up: Patients were evaluated 2 and 12 months after surgery. Postoperative examinations were performed by a gynecologist other than the operating surgeon if possible.

Endpoints: Primary outcome: Composite measure of (a) ≤ Stage 1 prolapse of the anterior vaginal wall as per the Pelvic Organ Prolapse Quantification (POP-Q) system[2] and (b) negative response to the question "Do you experience a feeling of bulging or protrusion in the vaginal area?" Secondary outcomes: Individual components of the primary outcome, surgical complications, adverse events, and patient-reported urogenital distress and sexual function (based on responses to validated questionnaires).

RESULTS

- 12 months after surgery, a statistically significant higher proportion of women in the mesh group had achieved Stage 0 or Stage 1 bladder

prolapse and had a negative response to the question of feeling of bulge or protrusion in the vaginal area compared to the native tissue repair group (60.8% vs. 35.5%).
- Complications and adverse events were more common in the mesh repair group, although none of the differences reached statistical significance of $p < 0.05$.
  - Bladder perforation rate was 3.5% in the mesh repair group and 0.5% in the traditional anterior repair group.
  - Intraoperative hemorrhage (>500mL) was more common in the mesh group than the native tissue group (2.7% vs. 0%).
  - Inguinal pain was more common during postoperative hospital stay in the mesh group than the native tissue group (2.5% vs. 0%).
  - Voiding dysfunction was more common during postoperative hospital stay in the mesh group than the native tissue group (8.0% vs. 3.2%).
- 3.2% of the mesh repair group versus 0% in the native repair group required surgical management of mesh exposure during the initial 12 months after surgery. This difference was statistically significant at $p = 0.05$.

Table 35.1. SUMMARY OF KEY FINDINGS

Successful Composite Primary Outcome (Anatomic and Symptomatic)	Native Tissue Colporrhaphy Group (%)	Mesh-augmented Repair Group (%)
2 months postoperative[a]	49.4	72.6
1 year postoperative*	34.5	60.8
Complications (within 2 months)		
Bladder perforation	3.5	0.5
Intraoperative hemorrhage	2.7	0
Inguinal pain	2.5	0
Voiding dysfunction	8.0	3.2
Complications (within 12 months)		
Mesh erosion requiring surgical repair[a]	3.2	0

[a]Difference is statistically significant ($p < 0.05$).

Criticisms and Limitations: First, this study only provides data for anterior vaginal wall prolapse and does not apply to those with apically dependent vaginal prolapse.

Second, the objective criteria for success (achieving Stage 0 or Stage 1 descent) is more stringent than current recommended definitions of successful prolapse surgery outcomes, which typically includes clinically relevant improvement; more recent studies define success as lack of patient symptoms and prolapse above the hymen (i.e., Stage 2 or less).

Third, this study reports a short follow-up period (12 months); other studies have demonstrated that mesh complications can present beyond 1 year.

Other Relevant Studies and Information:

- Several other studies have evaluated transvaginal mesh for pelvic organ prolapse and support the conclusion that mesh demonstrates improved anatomic outcomes, but with a higher rate of adverse events than repair with native tissue.[3,4,5] The improvement is particularly pronounced with an updated definition of "success" as absence of prolapse beyond the hymen without symptoms of prolapse, which correlates most closely to patients' self-reported assessment of a procedure as successful.[6]
- The Food and Drug Administration (FDA) ordered the immediate cessation of distribution of all transvaginal mesh for the repair of anterior compartment prolapse in April 2019.[7,8] The FDA stated this decision was based on insufficient evidence of efficacy and safety compared to native tissue repair.
- The FDA's announcement also stated specifically that patients who had already had transvaginal mesh placement for surgical repair of prolapse should continue with annual and routine care and that no additional action was necessary if patients were not having complications or issues with the mesh.[9]
- The American College of Obstetricians and Gynecologists and the American Urogynecologic Society have issued recommendations that existing mesh should be left in place in asymptomatic patients.[10]

Summary and Implications: This study suggests that transvaginal mesh repair of anterior compartment prolapse is associated with lower rates of objective and subjective prolapse symptoms 12 months after surgery compared with native tissue repair. However, these benefits come at the expense of greater risks, such as mesh erosion and mesh-associated pelvic pain.

CLINICAL CASE

Case History

A 67-year old G4P4 presents several years after surgical repair of anterior vaginal prolapse with transvaginal mesh. The patient takes metformin for her well-controlled type II diabetes mellitus, vaginal estrogen for vulvovaginal atrophy, and 81mg of aspirin and a calcium supplement daily. She is currently sexually active and has no pain with vaginal intercourse, nor does she have generalized pelvic pain. Physical exam demonstrates no significant recurrence of her prolapse, and her anterior, posterior, and apical compartments of the vagina are at least 1cm above the hymen. She has no other surgical history. The patient wants to know if she should have her vaginal mesh removed based on the FDA press release that she has seen mentioned in several news articles. How do you counsel this patient?

Suggested Answer

This patient should be offered reassurance that she does not need to have her mesh removed as she is not currently experiencing any complications related to the mesh and has not had a recurrence of her prolapse. She should be directed to the FDA News release[8] relating to transvaginally placed mesh, which again specifically states that patients do not need their mesh removed if they are satisfied with their repair and they are not experiencing any complications such as bleeding, erosions, or recurrent infections.

As already discussed, long-term rates of mesh complications requiring surgical intervention are limited, which was part of the FDA's justification halting the distribution of transvaginal mesh. However, in the absence of complication, surgical removal of the mesh implant is not recommended. Conversely, if the patient were to present with issues consistent with a mesh complication, prolapse recurrence, evaluation by an appropriately trained and experienced subspecialist would be indicated.

References

1. Altman D, Väyrynen T, Engh ME, Axelsen S, Falconer C, Nordic Transvaginal Mesh Group. Anterior colporrhaphy versus transvaginal mesh for pelvic-organ prolapse. *N Engl J Med.* 2011 May 12;364(19):1826–1836. doi:10.1056/NEJMoa1009521. Erratum in: *N Engl J Med.* 2013 Jan 24;368(4):394.
2. Persu C, Chapple CR, Cauni V, Gutue S, Geavlete P. Pelvic Organ Prolapse Quantification System (POP-Q)—a new era in pelvic prolapse staging. *J Med Life.* 2011;4(1):75–81.

3. Maher C, Feiner B, Baessler K, Schmid C. Surgical management of pelvic organ prolapse in women. *Cochrane Database Sys Rev.* 2013;4:CD004014. https://doi.org/10.1002/14651858.CD004014.pub5.

4. Dias, MM., de A Castro R, Bortolini ATM, Delroy CA, Martins PCF, Manoel, Girão JBC, Sartori MGF. Two-years results of native tissue versus vaginal mesh repair in the treatment of anterior prolapse according to different success criteria: a randomized controlled trial. *Neurourol Urodynam.* 2016;35(4):509–514. https://doi.org/10.1002/nau.22740.

5. Vollebregt A, Fischer K, Gietelink D, van der Vaart CH. Primary surgical repair of anterior vaginal prolapse: a randomised trial comparing anatomical and functional outcome between anterior colporrhaphy and trocar-guided transobturator anterior mesh. *BJOG.* 2011;118(12):1518–1527. https://doi.org/10.1111/j.1471-0528.2011.03082.x.

6. Barber MD, Brubaker L, Nygaard I, et al. Defining success after surgery for pelvic organ prolapse. *Obstet Gynecol.* 2009;114:600–609.

7. Chmielewski L, Walters MD, Weber AM, Barber MD. Reanalysis of a randomized trial of 3 techniques of anterior colporrhaphy using clinically relevant definitions of success. *Am J Obstet Gynecol.* 2011;205(1):69.e1–8.

8. FDA News Release. FDA takes action to protect women's health, orders manufacturers of surgical mesh intended for transvaginal repair of pelvic organ prolapse to stop selling all devices. https://www.fda.gov/news-events/press-announcements/fda-takes-action-protect-womens-health-orders-manufacturers-surgical-mesh-intended-transvaginal

9. FDA Statement on urogynecologic surgical mesh implants. https://www.fda.gov/medical-devices/implants-and-prosthetics/urogynecologic-surgical-mesh-implants

10. Management of mesh and graft complications in gynecologic surgery. Committee Opinion No. 694. American College of Obstetricians and Gynecologists. *Obstet Gynecol.* 2017;129:e102–e108

36

Preoperative Urodynamics Testing in Stress Urinary Incontinence

The VALUE Trial

LINDA BURKETT AND MEGAN BRADLEY

"Basic office assessment for women with uncomplicated stress-predominant urinary incontinence, who have stress incontinence on office evaluation, is noninferior to preoperative evaluation that also includes urodynamic testing."

—THE VALUE INVESTIGATORS[1]

Research Question: Do women with clinically demonstrable stress urinary incontinence (SUI) benefit from urodynamic testing prior to surgical management?[1]

Funding: National Institute of Diabetes and Digestive and Kidney Disease and the Eunice Kennedy Shriver National Institute of Child Health and Human Development

Year Study Began: 2008

Year Study Published: 2012

Study Location: 11 academic medical centers in the United States

Who Was Studied: Women over the age of 21 desiring surgical management for SUI, with symptoms lasting for at least 3 months. Clinically women had urethral hypermobility and leakage by provocative stress test (observed loss of urine with cough or valsalva at any bladder volume).[2] In addition, only women with post-void residual urine volume (PVR) < 150 ml and normal urinalysis were eligible.

Who Was Excluded: Women with pelvic organ prolapse > Stage II Pelvic Organ Prolapse Quantification (POP-Q) (anterior or apical leading edge 1cm past hymen), a history of any incontinence surgery, pelvic surgery in the last 3 months, pelvic radiation, or active gynecologic malignancy.

How Many Patients: 630

Study Overview: See Figure 36.1

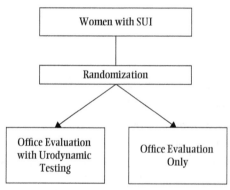

Figure 36.1. Study overview: the VALUE Trial

Study Intervention: Patients were randomized to receive simple office evaluation only or simple office evaluation with preoperative urodynamics (UDS) testing prior to surgical treatment for SUI. Planned procedures included retropubic or transobturator midurethral sling, mini-sling, traditional sling, retropubic urethropexy, or urethral bulking.

Follow-Up: 12 months

Endpoints: Primary outcome: Treatment success (composite outcome) reduction in the score on the Urogenital Distress Inventory of >70% from baseline to 12 months postoperatively and response of Patient Global Impression of Improvement of "much better" or "very much better" at 12 months after surgery. Secondary outcomes: Surgical success assessed by provocative stress test with 300ml bladder fill and other patient symptom questionnaires.

RESULTS

- A basic office evaluation was noninferior to a basic office evaluation with the addition of UDS.
- Treatment success and patient symptoms (composite primary outcome) were not significantly different in office evaluation only (77.2%) or with the addition of UDS (76.9%).
- Surgical treatment success (negative provocative stress test at 12 months) was not different between office evaluation only (72.9%) versus UDS (69.4%) groups, see Table 36.1.
- Overall, the distribution of surgical treatment types was equal between groups, with approximately 93% of patients undergoing a mid-urethral sling.

Table 36.1. SUMMARY OF VALUE TRIAL KEY FINDINGS

12-Month Follow-Up	Office Evaluation Only (%)	UDS + Office Evaluation (%)
Treatment Success	77.2	76.9
Surgical Success	72.9	69.4

Abbreviation: UDS, preoperative urodynamics.

Criticisms and Limitations: It is important to note that the scope of this study was limited to assessment of patients with only uncomplicated and symptomatic SUI. Urodynamics testing does provide diagnostic information in patients with complex voiding dysfunction, and therefore it continues to have an important role in clinical practice.

All practices and surgeons were fellowship trained in Uro Gynecology decreasing generalizability to providers who may not have the same level of experience and training in evaluation of complex urinary incontinence.

Other Relevant Studies and Information:

- The AUA/SUFU 2012 guidelines on urodynamics studies in adults states that "clinicians may perform multi-channel urodynamics in patients with both symptoms and physical findings of stress incontinence who are considering invasive, potentially morbid or irreversible treatments" with grade C evidence.[3]

- However, the AUA/SUFU guidelines do support that for uncomplicated patients, with demonstrable stress incontinence, UDS is not necessary. Uncomplicated patients are defined as those without medical comorbidities, prior pelvic surgery, neurologic symptoms, prolapse, or other dysfunctional urinary complaints.[3]
- A secondary analysis of the VALUE data was completed evaluating the influence of preoperative urodynamic studies results on diagnoses and treatment plans. This analysis was meant to address concerns about UDS changing patient surgical or treatment plans. UDS testing did change the clinical diagnoses in 57% of patients; however, it only resulted in a change in treatment plan on rare occasions. Treatment plans were adjusted in 14% of patients to include additional nonsurgical treatment postoperatively, 1.4% canceled surgery, and 5.4% had the type of SUI surgery changed. Yet, these changes did not result in improved treatment outcomes.[4,5]

Summary and Implications: This study demonstrated that preoperative urodynamics testing, which is costly, uncomfortable, and time consuming, does not result in an improvement in surgical or symptomatic outcomes for uncomplicated SUI. Further studies have also showed that UDS may change the preoperative diagnoses but not treatment plan, and that UDS findings have not been shown to be predictive of treatment failure. The results of this study suggest that UDS testing should only be considered in patients with complicated SUI.

CLINICAL CASE

Case History

A 56-year-old postmenopausal female presents to clinic with the complaint of urinary incontinence. She reports having to wear 2 to 3 pads per day with very bothersome symptoms. She reports leakage with laugh, cough, and sneeze for over 2 years. She denies symptoms of urinary urgency or frequency. She denies history of pelvic surgery or malignancy. Her past medical history is only significant for hypertension and hypothyroidism. On examination, she has a post-void residual of 50ml. She does not have pelvic organ prolapse with mild vaginal atrophy noted. She has positive cough stress test with 50ml in her bladder. Her urinalysis was normal. She is interested in definitive surgical options. What are the next steps in preoperative management for this patient?

Suggested Answer

This patient has uncomplicated stress urinary incontinence and does not meet criteria for urodynamic testing per study findings and the AUA/SUFU guidelines on urodynamics in adults.[3] She does not have prior surgeries, medical comorbidities, or other symptoms of voiding dysfunction. She should complete preoperative counseling regarding surgical options without further diagnostic testing.

References

1. Nager CW, Brubaker L, Litman HJ, et al. A randomized trial of urodynamic testing before stress-incontinence surgery. *N Engl J Med.* 2012;366(21):1987–1997.
2. Nager CW, Brubaker L, Daneshgari F, et al. Design of the Value of Urodynamic Evaluation (ValUE) trial: a non-inferiority randomized trial of preoperative urodynamic investigations. *Contemp Clin Trials.* 2009;30(6):531–539.
3. Winters JC, Dmochowski RR, Goldman HB, et al. Urodynamic studies in adults: AUA/SUFU guideline. *J Urol.* 2012;188(6 Suppl):2464–2472.
4. Sirls LT, Richter HE, Litman HJ, et al. The effect of urodynamic testing on clinical diagnosis, treatment plan and outcomes in women undergoing stress urinary incontinence surgery. *J Urol.* 2013;189(1):204–209.
5. Norton PA, Nager CW, Brubaker L, et al. The cost of preoperative urodynamics: a secondary analysis of the ValUE trial. *Neurourol Urodyn.* 2016;35(1):81–84.

37

A Midurethral Sling to Reduce Incontinence After Vaginal Repair

The OPUS Trial

DEEPALI MAHESHWARI AND ELLEN SOLOMON

"Adding a midurethral sling at the time of vaginal-prolapse surgery in women without preoperative symptoms of stress urinary incontinence reduces the likelihood of urinary incontinence at 3-12 months after surgery but increase the likelihood of adverse events."
—THE OPUS INVESTIGATORS[1]

Research Question: Should patients without preoperative stress urinary incontinence receive a midurethral sling at the time of prolapse repair to reduce the risk of postoperative stress urinary incontinence (SUI)?

Funding: Eunice Kennedy Shriver National Institute of Child Health and Human Development and the National Institutes of Health Office of Research on Women's Health

Year Study Began: 2007

Year Study Published: 2012

Study Location: 7 clinical sites across the United States

Who Was Studied: Women who were planning to undergo vaginal prolapse surgery who reported the symptom of feeling or seeing a vaginal bulge but reported no symptoms of SUI, which was defined as a positive response to specific questions regarding stress incontinence on the Pelvic Floor Distress Inventory.

Who Was Excluded: Women who had undergone previous sling placement, were receiving treatment for SUI, for whom a sling was contraindicated, were planning pregnancy within a year post-surgery, or had 2 or more hospitalizations for medical illnesses in the previous year.

How Many Patients: 337

Study Overview: See Figure 37.1

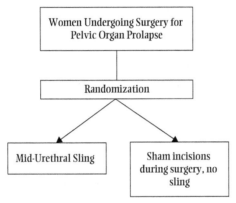

Figure 37.1. Study overview: the OPUS Trial

Study Intervention: Women in the intervention group received a prophylactic retropubic midurethral sling (Gynecare TVT, Ethicon) at the time of vaginal prolapse surgery. These women did not have any pre-existing stress urinary incontinence.

Women in the control group received two 1cm suprapubic sham incisions, which were designed to mimic sling incisions.

Follow-Up: 3, 6, and 12 months consisting of medical history taking, survey administration, assessment of prolapse, cough stress test, urinalysis, and measurement of postvoid residual volume

Endpoints: Primary outcome: Urinary incontinence (stress, urge, or mixed) at 3 months and urinary incontinence at 12 months. Secondary outcomes: Measures of incontinence and quality of life (Pelvic Floor Distress Inventory, Pelvic Organ Prolapse/Urinary Incontinence Sexual Function Questionnaire Short Form, visual analogue pain scale), serious adverse events, expected complications, and unexpected non-serious adverse events

RESULTS

- At 12 months, the sling group had lower rates of urinary incontinence as compared to those in the sham group (27.3% vs. 43%, see Table 37.1). Patients in the sling group also had a greater reduction in baseline urinary symptoms as measured on the Pelvic Floor Distress Inventory.
- The number needed to treat with a sling to prevent 1 case of urinary incontinence or treatment of incontinence at 3 months was 3.9 and at 12 months was 6.3.
- There were no significant differences between groups with respect to generic health, pelvic-floor symptoms, effect on quality of life, sexual function, pain, or rates of serious or unexpected adverse events.
- Rates of bladder perforation, urinary tract infection, major bleeding complications, and incomplete bladder emptying at time of surgery and for the subsequent 6 weeks were all higher in the sling group than in the control group. There were no mesh erosions.
- In a cohort of women who declined randomized, those who chose sling treatment had lower rates of urinary incontinence at similar rates to the intervention group; however, the findings were not statistically significant.

Table 37.1. SUMMARY OF KEY FINDINGS

	Sling % ($n = 165$)	Control % ($n = 172$)	*p*-value
3-month urinary incontinence rate	23.6	49.4	<0.001
12-month urinary incontinence rate	27.3	43	<0.001

Criticisms and Limitations: This study is limited by the 12-month follow-up duration; results should not be extrapolated beyond that period of time. It is also noted that the type of apical suspension or anterior repair may have impacted success of the operation, but this study was not powered to study those differences.

Other Relevant Studies and Information:

- The CARE (Colpopexy and Urinary Reduction Efforts) trial,[2] which was carried out a decade prior, found that the addition of surgical treatment for SUI (the Burch colposuspension) at the time of abdominal prolapse surgery reduced the incidence of postoperative SUI. The results of the OPUS trial support that finding, but instead utilize the midurethral sling procedure, which is less morbid and requires less operative time.

- The data from this trial was used to create a calculator to predict the risk of de novo SUI after vaginal pelvic prolapse surgery.[3] Factors include age, BMI, number of vaginal births, diagnosis of diabetes, urge urinary leakage, and preoperative stress test result. It is validated and can be found at: http://riskcalc.org/FemalePelvicMedicineandReconstructive Surgery/ or in mobile app form at www.augs.org/augs-now-app.

- The American College of Obstetricians and Gynecologists and American Urogynecologic Society guidelines suggest that patients undergoing surgery for pelvic organ prolapse who do not have preoperative symptoms of stress incontinence should be counseled regarding their risk for post-operative SUI without a prophylactic sling procedure, but must be informed regarding the increased risk for adverse outcomes associated with the additional procedure.[4]

Summary and Implications: The OPUS trial demonstrated that, among women undergoing a vaginal prolapse repair, there was a decrease in postoperative urinary incontinence and treatment for urinary incontinence at 3 and 12 months in women who received a prophylactic sling at the time of the repair. There was a higher rate of adverse effects with sling placement, however, including bladder perforation during sling placement, urinary tract infection, incomplete bladder emptying, and major bleeding or vascular complication.

CLINICAL CASE: A MIDURETHRAL SLING AT THE TIME OF VAGINAL PROLAPSE SURGERY

Case History

A 63-year-old woman with symptomatic pelvic organ prolapse presents for surgical counseling. She denies any symptoms of stress or urge urinary incontinence. A preoperative cough stress test with the prolapse reduction is negative. She would like to proceed with a vaginal hysterectomy, uterosacral ligament suspension, and anterior repair. Based on the results of the OPUS trial, how should she be counseled?

Suggested Answer

Current guidelines recommend a nuanced counseling regarding prophylactic surgery for SUI at the time of prolapse surgery. This patient should be counseled that nearly half of women who do not have a concurrent midurethral sling at the time of prolapse surgery develop de novo stress urinary incontinence after surgery. A midurethral sling at the time of her prolapse surgery may reduce her risk of having urinary incontinence by 40% as compared to women who do not have a sling placed at the time of surgery. The sling can be placed as a subsequent surgical procedure with additional surgical and anesthetic risk. Her counseling should also include that the addition of a sling is associated with an increased risk of adverse events including bladder perforation, urinary tract infection, bleeding, and incomplete bladder emptying.

References

1. Wei JT, Nygaard I, Richter HE, Nager CW, Barber MD, Kenton K, Amundsen CL, Schaffer J, Meikle SF, Spino C; Pelvic Floor Disorders Network. A midurethral sling to reduce incontinence after vaginal prolapse repair. *N Engl J Med.* 2012 Jun 21;366(25):2358–2367.

2. Brubaker L, Cundiff GW, Fine P, et al. Abdominal sacrocolpopexy with Burch colpopsuspension to reduce urinary stress incontinence. *N Engl J Med.* 2006;354(15):1557–1566.

3. Jelovsek JE, Chagin K, Brubaker L, Rogers RG, Richter HE, Arya L, Barber MD, Shepherd JP, Nolen TL, Norton P, Sung V, Menefee S, Siddiqui N, Meikle SF, Kattan MW, Pelvic Floor Disorders Network. A model for predicting the risk of de novo stress urinary incontinence in women undergoing pelvic organ prolapse surgery. *Obstet Gynecol.* 2014;123(2 Pt 1):279–287.

4. Committee on Practice Bulletins—Gynecology and the American Urogynecologic Society. ACOG Practice Bulletin No. 155: urinary incontinence in women. *Obstet Gynecol.* 2015 Nov; 126(5):e66–e81.

38

Uterine-Artery Embolization Versus Surgery for Symptomatic Uterine Fibroids

KRISTEN PEPIN AND SARAH L. COHEN

"Our study makes clear that the choice between surgery and uterine-artery embolization for symptomatic fibroids involves tradeoffs."
—THE REST INVESTIGATORS[1]

Research Question: How does quality of life following uterine artery embolization compare to that associated with surgical treatment of symptomatic uterine fibroids?

Funding: Chief Scientist Office of the Scottish Executive, William Cooke Europe, Cordis, Biocompatibles

Year Study Began: 2000

Year Study Published: 2007

Location: 27 Hospitals in the United Kingdom

Who Was Studied: Adult women with 1 or more fibroids at least 2cm in diameter. To be included, the fibroids had to be visible on magnetic resonance imaging (MRI), symptomatic (causing menorrhagia, pelvic pain, or pressure), and appropriate for surgical intervention as determined by the treating physician.

Who Was Excluded: Patients in whom MRI or surgery was contraindicated, those with iodinated contrast media allergy, those with subserosal pedunculated fibroids, recent or current pelvic inflammatory disease, and pregnant patients

How Many Patients: 157

Study Overview: See Figure 38.1

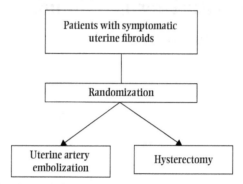

Figure 38.1. Study overview: the REST Trial

Study Intervention: Patients were randomized to either surgery or embolization. Patients in the surgery group underwent hysterectomy or myomectomy, depending on their future fertility goals. All surgeries were performed using an abdominal laparotomy. The technique for embolization was not specified, but both uterine arteries had to be embolized and the particle size of the embolic agent was standardized to 500–710 μm.

Follow-Up: 12 months for the primary and the majority of secondary outcomes; major adverse events and subsequent interventions were reported over the length of the study with a maximum follow-up of 58 months

Endpoints: Primary outcome was quality of life at 1-year post-procedure as measured by a validated quality of life survey called the Medical Outcomes Study 36-Item Short-Form General Health Survey (SF-36, score ranging from 0 to 100 with higher scores indicating higher functioning). Secondary outcomes were score on EuroQol-5D questionnaire (a validated survey), time to resumption of usual activities, patient satisfaction score, pain score at 24 hours post-procedure, occurrence of complications, and treatment failure (need for hysterectomy or repeat embolization).

RESULTS

- At 1 month post-procedure, the patients in the uterine artery embolization group had a statistically significantly improvement in scores for physical and social function. Patients in the embolization group had a faster resumption of normal activities than those in the surgery group.
- Patients in the surgical group had lower symptom scores at 1 and 12 months after hysterectomy or myomectomy.
- Major complications occurred in 15% of patients in the embolization group and 20% of women in the surgery group. Minor complications occurred in 34% of patients in the embolization group and 20% of women in the surgery group. Patients in the surgical group had higher pain scores during the first 24 hours after their procedure.
- At 12 months, there was no difference in the SF-36 scores between the surgery group and the uterine artery embolization group.
- Among women treated with uterine artery embolization, 20% required an additional invasive procedure for continued or recurrent symptoms.
- Uterine artery embolization was associated with lower total costs than surgery, driven primarily by lower inpatient costs. See Table 38.1.

Table 38.1. SUMMARY OF FINDINGS

Measure	Embolization Group	Surgery Group	p-value
SF-36 score of Physical Function at 12 months post-procedure	92 ± 14	89 ± 20	0.85
SF-36 score of Social Function at 12 months post-procedure	84 ± 23	87 ± 26	0.35
Pain score at 24 hours post-procedure	3.0 ± 2.1	4.6 ± 2.3	<0.001
Median Duration of Hospitalization in Days	1	5	<0.001
Median Days of Missed Work	20	62	<0.001
Minor Complications within 12 months	36 (34%)	10 (20%)	0.047
Major Complications within 12 months	16 (15%)	10 (20%)	0.22
Fibroid Symptom Score at 12 month (High score = fewer symptoms)	3.6 ± 2.0	4. 3 ± 1.7	0.03
Treatment failure within 12 months	21 (20%)	1 (2%)	Not reported

Abbreviation: SF-36, Short-Form General Health Survey.

Criticisms and Limitations: The study included only patients undergoing abdominal surgical procedures and does not provide a comparison between uterine-artery embolization and minimally invasive surgical approaches. Additionally, only a small number of patients in the surgery group underwent myomectomy (8 patients), making it difficult to use this study to compare uterine preserving interventions.

Other Relevant Studies and Information:

- Several additional studies have shown no difference in the quality of life after uterine artery embolization vs. surgery.[2–4]
- In a Cochrane review and meta-analysis published in 2014, data from 7 randomized controlled trials (including REST) comparing uterine artery embolization and surgical management and involving a total of 793 patients found that uterine artery embolization was associated with shorter hospital stays and faster return to normal activities but also a higher rate of minor complications and reintervention (15%–32% vs. 7% in the surgery group).[5–8]
- According to the American College of Obstetricians and Gynecologists, uterine artery embolization is a safe option for appropriately selected women who wish to avoid hysterectomy.[8]

Summary and Implications: For the treatment of symptomatic uterine fibroids, uterine-artery embolization and surgery (abdominal myomectomy or hysterectomy) result in similar quality of life scores at 1 year after the procedure. Patients undergoing uterine-artery embolization have lower pain scores 24 hours post-procedure, stay in the hospital less time, and get back to work faster but have a reintervention rate of 20% within the first year. Rates of major and minor complications between uterine-artery embolization and surgery are comparable.

CLINICAL CASE: UTERINE ARTERY EMBOLIZATION VERSUS SURGERY FOR SYMPTOMATIC UTERINE FIBROIDS

Case History

A 45-year-old Gravida 3 Para 2 with menorrhagia and pelvic bulk symptoms is noted to have an 8cm posterior intramural fibroid on pelvic ultrasound. She has failed medical management of her menorrhagia. Based on the results of the

REST trial, how would you counsel the patient about the risks and benefits of uterine-artery embolization versus abdominal hysterectomy?

Suggested Answer

The REST trial showed that patients treated for symptomatic uterine fibroids had with uterine-artery embolization and surgery had the same quality of life 1 year after the procedure. Your patient should know that if choosing uterine-artery embolization, she will likely have less pain and a shorter hospital stay and will get back to work faster. However, she has a 20% chance of needing to an additional invasive procedure (such as hysterectomy) for a treatment failure. Additionally, although it was not directly addressed in this trial, minimally invasive surgical treatments for fibroids can provide the dual benefits of curative intent and optimized recovery parameters. She should understand that rates of complications, both major and minor, are similar for both procedures.

References

1. Edwards RD, Moss JG, Lumsden MA, Wu O, Murray LS, Twaddle S, Murray GD. Uterine-artery embolization versus surgery for symptomatic uterine fibroids. *N Eng J Med.* 2007;356 (4):360–370. doi:10.1056/NEJMoa062003.

2. Jun F, Yamin L, Xinli X, Zhe L, Min Z, Bo Z, Wenli G. Uterine artery embolization versus surgery for symptomatic uterine fibroids: a randomized controlled trial and a meta-analysis of the literature. *Arch Gynecol Obstet.* 2012;285:1407–1413.

3. Manyonda IT, Bratby M, Horst JS, Banu N, Gorti M, Belli A-M. Uterine artery embolization versus myomectomy: impact on quality of life—results of the FUME (Fibroids of the Uterus: Myomectomy versus Embolization) trial. *Cardiovasc Interven Radiol.* 2012;35(3):530–536.

4. Ruuskanen A, Hippelainen M, Sipola P, Manninen H. Uterine artery embolisation versus hysterectomy for leiomyomas: primary and 2-year follow-up results of a randomised prospective clinical trial. *Eur Radiol.* 2010;20(10):2524–2532.

5. Gupta JK, Sinha A, Lumsden MA, Hickey M. Uterine artery embolization for symptomatic uterine fibroids. *Cochrane Database Sys Rev.* 2014;12:CD005073.

6. Mara M, Maskova J, Fucikova Z, Kuzel D, Belsan T, Sosna O. Midterm clinical and first reproductive results of a randomized controlled trial comparing uterine fibroid embolization and myomectomy. *Cardiovasc Interven Radiol.* 2008;31:73–85.

7. Pinto I, Chimeno P, Romo L, Haya J, De la Cal M, Bajo J. Uterine fibroids: uterine artery embolization versus abdominal hysterectomy for treatment. A prospective randomized and controlled trial. *Radiology.* 2003;226(2):425–431.

8. American College of Obstetricians and Gynecologists. ACOG practice bulletin. Alternatives to hysterectomy in the management of leiomyomas. *Obstet Gynecol.* 2008;112(2 Pt 1):387–400.

39

Robotic-Assisted Versus Laparoscopic Hysterectomy Among Women With Benign Gynecologic Disease

CHETNA ARORA AND ARNOLD P. ADVINCULA

"From a public health standpoint, defining subsets of patients with benign gynecologic disorders who derive benefit from robotic hysterectomy, reducing the cost of robotic instrumentation, and developing initiatives to promote laparoscopic hysterectomy are warranted."

—JD WRIGHT ET AL.[1]

Research Question: Is the increase in the uptake of the robotic-assisted approach for hysterectomy associated with more costs and complications?

Funding: This study was supported in part by a grant from the National Cancer Institute (R01CA134964).

Study Years: 2007–2010

Publication Year: 2013

Study Location: 441 hospitals across the United States

Who Was Studied: Women 18 years or older who underwent a hysterectomy for a benign disorder

Who Was Excluded: Women undergoing surgery for gynecologic malignancy

How Many Patients: 264,758

Study Overview: See Figure 39.1

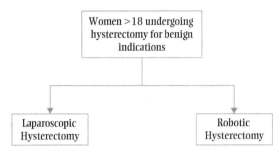

Figure 39.1. Study overview

Study Intervention: The study evaluated outcomes according to route of surgery.

Follow-Up: Not applicable

Endpoints: Primary outcome: Uptake of and factors associated with utilization of robotically assisted hysterectomy. Secondary outcome: Complications, transfusion, reoperation, length of stay, death, and cost for women who underwent robotic hysterectomy compared to both laparoscopic and abdominal hysterectomy.

RESULTS

- Robotic-assisted hysterectomy rate increased over the study interval from 0.5% to 9.5% whereas vaginal and abdominal hysterectomy routes decreased. In institutions where the robotic approach was not available, the rates of laparoscopic hysterectomy increased with proportional decreases in the alternative routes.
- After the introduction of robotic-assisted hysterectomy at a given hospital, uptake was rapid; in these hospitals, robotic-assisted hysterectomy accounted for 22.4% of all hysterectomies within 3 years.
- The most common indication for the use of robotic technology was abnormal uterine bleeding.

- The rates of intraoperative complications between the robotic-assisted and laparoscopic hysterectomy groups (2.5% vs. 2.4%; relative risk [RR] 1.05; 95% confidence interval [CI] 0.75–1.47), surgical site complications (1.7% vs. 2.0%; RR 0.85; 95% CI 0.64–1.13), and medical complications (1.6% vs. 1.2%; RR 1.35; 95% CI 0.97–1.88) were similar between the groups. In a propensity score–matched analysis, the overall complication rates were similar for robotic-assisted and laparoscopic hysterectomy (5.5% vs. 5.3%; RR 1.03; 95% CI 0.86–1.24). See Table 39.1.
- Cost was defined as fixed costs (unchanged by patient volume and include purchase of robotic platform), variable costs (i.e., disposable instrumentation and supplies), and total costs. Robotic surgery was associated with $2189 (95% CI, $2073–$2377) increased total costs, $962 (95% CI, $878– $1047) increased fixed costs, and $1207 (95% CI, $1110–$1304) increased variable costs compared with laparoscopic surgery. See Table 39.1.

Table 39.1. OUTCOMES AND COST OF LAPAROSCOPIC VERSUS ROBOTIC HYSTERECTOMY

	Laparoscopic Hysterectomy n = 4971 (%)	Robotic Hysterectomy n = 4971 (%)	*p*-value
Complications	264 (5.3)	271 (5.5)	0.76
Total cost, $	6679	8868	<.001
Fixed cost, $	3040	4002	<.001
Variable cost, $	3493	4700	<.001

- Sensitivity analyses on the relationship between the cost of robotic-assisted hysterectomy and volume showed that, as the volume of robotic cases increased, physician costs per procedure increased while hospital operational costs decreased.

Criticisms and Limitations: The study did not include important demographic and clinical factors such as body mass index (BMI), uterine weight, prior surgical history, operative time, stage of endometriosis, or number, size, and location of fibroids, which likely influenced route of surgery.

The analysis of cost included only direct hospital costs incurred for the procedure itself. Thus the cost estimates in this analysis may not take into account other costs, such as length of inpatient stay or recovery time.

This study was published early in the evolution of robotic technology and robotic implementation; the outcomes might be different if this study were to be repeated.

Other Relevant Studies and Information:

- Other studies have shown that robotic-assisted hysterectomy is associated with improved outcomes when compared to all alternative routes when performed by high-volume gynecologic surgeons. Examples of improved outcomes include lower intraoperative and postoperative complication rates, decreased conversion rates, and lower 30-day readmission rates all with significant downstream cost savings.[1-7]
- More complicated pathology such as increasing uterine weight or patient obesity can significantly increase operative times and, as a result, cost. When more complex pathology is encountered, laparoscopic surgery is associated with comparatively longer operative times compared to robotic surgery.[5,8]

The American Association of Gynecologic Laparoscopists (AAGL) recommends that most benign hysterectomies should be performed either vaginally or laparoscopically. The American College of Obstetricians and Gynecologists advocates for continued study to identify those patients who would specifically benefit from a robot-assisted approach.[9,10]

Summary and Implications: Robotic-assisted hysterectomy for benign disease underwent a rapid uptake after introduction. It has similar rates of complications to laparoscopic hysterectomy but a higher overall cost.

CLINICAL CASE

Case History

A 45-year-old morbidly-obese female presents to clinic with abnormal uterine bleeding and pelvic pressure likely due to multiple uterine fibroids. Exam shows a 20-week myomatous uterus. She has failed medical management, hemoglobin is 8.5, and she now desires definitive management by means of a hysterectomy. Her provider favors an open approach. He does not perform robotic-assisted hysterectomies and feels the patient is not a candidate for conventional laparoscopic surgery given the fibroid burden.

Which route of surgery is preferred for hysterectomy in this patient?
Should this provider refer the patient to someone trained in robotic surgery?

Suggested Answer

Patients with increasing obesity, medical comorbidities, and significant uterine pathology may be candidates for consideration for the robotic approach when an open approach would have otherwise been the alternative. For the patient with the lower BMI and smaller uterus, she should first be determined for candidacy of a vaginal approach and then consideration of the laparoscopic route if not feasible. With the patient with the higher BMI and larger uterus, she may benefit from the robotic approach if vaginal or other laparoscopic approaches are not appropriate due to increasing overall complexity. Given the morbidity of an open approach in a patient with Class III obesity and preoperative anemia, if a minimally-invasive option is at all feasible, it should be preferred. This patient should be referred to a gynecologic surgeon trained in robotics for a second opinion on candidacy for this approach as needed. Ultimately, overall morbidity and cost can be mitigated by appropriately individualizing patient-centered care and route of surgery.

References

1. Wright JD, Ananth CV, Lewin SN, et al. Robotically assisted vs laparoscopic hysterectomy among women with benign gynecologic disease. *JAMA*. 2013;309(7):689–698. doi:10.1001/jama.2013.186
2. Lim PC, Crane JT, English EJ, et al. Multicenter analysis comparing robotic, open, laparoscopic, and vaginal hysterectomies performed by high-volume surgeons for benign indications. *Int J Gynecol Obstet*. 2016;133(3):359–364.
3. Five things patients and providers should question. Choosing Wisely—Promoting conversations between providers and patients. http://www.choosingwisely.org/societies/aagl/.
4. Martino MA, Berger EA, McFetridge JT, et al. A comparison of quality outcome measures in patients having a hysterectomy for benign disease: robotic vs. non-robotic approaches. *J Minim Invasive Gynecol*. 2014;21(3):389–393.
5. Lonnerfors C, Reynisson P, Persson J. A randomized trial comparing vaginal and laparoscopic hysterectomy vs robot-assisted hysterectomy. *J Minim Invasive Gynecol*. 2015;22(1):78–86.
6. Winter ML, Leu SY, Lagrew DC, Jr., Bustillo G. Cost comparison of robotic-assisted laparoscopic hysterectomy versus standard laparoscopic hysterectomy. *J Robot Surg*. 2015;9(4):269–275.
7. Jonsdottir GM, Jorgensen S, Cohen SL, et al. Increasing minimally invasive hysterectomy: effect on cost and complications. *Obstet Gynecol*. 2011;117(5):1142–1149.

8. Martinez-Maestre MA, Gambadauro P, Gonzalez-Cejudo C, Torrejon R. Total laparoscopic hysterectomy with and without robotic assistance: a prospective controlled study. *Surg Innov.* 2014;21(3):250–255.

9. AAGL Advancing Minimally Invasive Gynecology Worldwide. AAGL position statement: route of hysterectomy to treat benign uterine disease. *J Minim Invasive Gynecol.* 2011;18:1–3.

10. ACOG. Committee Opinion No. 628: robotic surgery in gynecology. *Obstet Gynecol.* 2015 Mar;125(3):760–767.

40

Endometrial Ablation Versus Hysterectomy

The STOP-DUB Trial

CHRISTINE HELOU AND MANDY YUNKER

"...both hysterectomy and endometrial ablation provide satisfactory results for women with dysfunctional uterine bleeding that has not responded to medical therapy. While almost one third of women having endometrial ablation will have reoperation within 5 years, hysterectomy is associated with more perioperative morbidity."
—STOP-DUB Research Group[1]

Research Question: Which is more effective: hysterectomy or endometrial ablation in women with dysfunctional uterine bleeding (DUB)?

Funding: Agency for Healthcare Research and Quality

Year Study Began: 1998

Year Study Published: 2007

Study Location: 33 clinical sites throughout the United States and Canada

Who Was Studied: Premenopausal women age >18 with DUB for at least 6 months and refractory to medical therapy for at least 3 months

Who Was Excluded: Pregnant women or those desiring future fertility, postmenopausal women, women with history of bilateral oophorectomy, fibroids, prior endometrial ablation, and women declining surgical treatment.[2]

How Many Patients: 237

Study Overview: See Figure 40.1

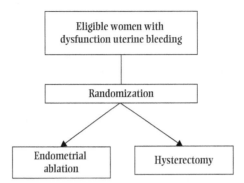

Figure 40.1 Study overview: the STOP-DUB Trial

Study Intervention: Patients qualifying for enrollment were randomized to either endometrial ablation (resectoscopic or vaporization) or hysterectomy (by any route). Randomized was stratified by clinical site and by age (<45 or 45+). Patients who were ineligible or declined randomized were placed in an observational arm to assess changes over time in symptoms and quality of life. These patients could opt for medical therapy if recommended by their physician or transfer to the randomized study arm if they became eligible over time.

Follow-Up: Up to 5 years

Endpoints: Primary outcomes: Resolution of patient's primary problem; effect on bleeding, pain, and fatigue at 12 months. Secondary outcomes: Effect on symptoms after 12 months, quality of life, activity, urinary incontinence, sexual function, surgical complications, and reoperation rates

---

RESULTS

- 80% of randomized patients reported excessive bleeding as the reason for seeking treatment.
- At 24 months postoperatively, both endometrial ablation and hysterectomy effectively resolved most patients' chief complaints (84.9% vs. 94.4%).
- There was a small but statistically significant difference in quality of life, with higher scores in the hysterectomy treatment group.

- Approximately 30% of patients initially undergoing endometrial ablation later underwent reoperation with hysterectomy (94%) or repeat ablation (6%).
- At 12 and 48 months, women treated with hysterectomy reported less pain overall. Women initially treated with ablation who then underwent reoperation initially reported more severe pain but then saw improvement after further surgery.
- Hysterectomy was more effective for addressing bleeding symptoms. Although volume of bleeding was usually improved with endometrial ablation, 15% of women receiving this treatment continued to report problems with frequency, predictability, and duration of bleeding.
- Hysterectomy was associated with 4 times ($n = 48$, 40.6%) more adverse events than among those undergoing ablation ($n = 12$, 10.9%) and 6 times more postoperative infections ($n = 19$, 16%) compared to those receiving ablation ($n = 3$, 2.7%).
- Patients in the observational arm ($n = 139$) were followed at least 6 months. Over the course of the study, 41 patients (29%) transferred from the observational arm to the surgical arm and were randomized to hysterectomy or ablation. See Table 40.1.

Table 40.1. SUMMARY OF STOP-DUB's KEY FINDINGS

Outcome	Ablation Group	Hysterectomy Group	*p*-value
Main Problem Solved at 24 Months	84.9%	94.4%	0.026
Severe Pelvic Pain at 24 Months	28.3%	6.5%	<0.01
Quality of Life Score at 6 Months	0.770	0.836	0.01
Adverse Events	10.9%	40.6%	NA

Criticisms and Limitations: The study was limited by small sample size due to slower-than-expected recruitment. In addition, the high rate of complications and adverse events limits the generalizability of this study. Women undergoing endometrial ablation were able to request concurrent tubal occlusion. It is possible that post-ablation sterilization syndrome contributed to overall failure of ablation in some patients. Finally, endometrial ablation in this study was carried out using a resectoscopic technique that is highly dependent on operator skill and has largely been replaced by nonresectoscopic global ablation methods. Thus the future applicability of resectoscopic data in comparison with hysterectomy may be limited.

Other Relevant Studies and Information:

- Other studies of endometrial ablation and hysterectomy, including a large Cochrane review, also showed a significant risk of reoperation in the group receiving endometrial ablation with similar reoperation rates of 23% to 36%.[3,4]
- Several similar randomized control trials showed no difference in quality of life between groups; however, these studies were underpowered to detect such a difference. Conversely, the few studies that found a difference in quality of life between treatment groups compared ablation specifically to minimally invasive routes of hysterectomy.[5]
- Several studies have examined the efficacy of endometrial ablation for DUB and the characteristics of patients most likely to have success with this method. Ahonkallio et al. found that women age >40 with heavy but regular menses did best.[6] Other studies confirmed that older patients (>45) tended to do better while African Americans, those with history of cesarean section or tubal ligation, chronic pelvic pain, obesity, and abnormal uterine findings on imaging (fibroids, polyps, thickened endometrial stripe) were more likely to fail treatment.[7–9]
- According to the American College of Obstetricians and Gynecologists, candidates for endometrial ablation include any premenopausal women with menorrhagia (or patient-perceived heavy menses) who do not desire future fertility and who have normal endometrial cavities.[10]

Summary and Implications: In patients with DUB unresponsive to medical management, both endometrial ablation and hysterectomy can lead to significant improvement of most symptoms, quality of life, and overall satisfaction. While hysterectomy is more effective at treating bleeding symptoms specifically, it is associated with longer recovery time, higher cost, and higher risk of complications. While the majority of patients that undergo endometrial ablation are satisfied with the outcome, almost one-third will require reoperation, often with hysterectomy. Once endometrial ablation is chosen, the surgeon and patient should consider patient-specific factors that impact the success of the procedure.

CLINICAL CASE: ENDOMETRIAL ABLATION VERSUS HYSTERECTOMY FOR DYSFUNCTIONAL UTERINE BLEEDING

Case History

A 40-year-old African American G4P4004 with history significant for chronic pelvic pain, obesity, and 3 prior cesarean sections presents to the office complaining of progressively worsening dysmenorrhea and heavy irregular menses. She has unsuccessfully been treated with oral contraceptives and a progesterone IUD in the past. She undergoes endometrial biopsy which shows disordered proliferative endometrium. She has had a tubal ligation and does not desire future fertility. She inquires if there are any surgical options to treat her bleeding problem. What would you recommend?

Suggested Answer

The information from the STOP-DUB trial could be used to counsel this patient about her surgical options. This trial showed that both endometrial ablation and hysterectomy are effective treatments for improving symptoms of DUB. While the majority of women who chose ablation are satisfied with the effect on their symptoms, a small percentage (~30%) will fail and require further surgery. Other studies related to the STOP-DUB trial could be used to assess how specific factors in this patient's history may affect the likelihood of success of either surgical treatment. Specifically, other studies have shown age <45, obesity, chronic pain, previous uterine surgery, structural intrauterine pathology, and African American race increase the risk of ablation failure.

Based on the findings of the STOP-DUB trial, endometrial ablation may be a reasonable choice for her if she desires a shorter recovery, seeks improvement of symptoms but not necessarily complete amenorrhea, or has medical comorbidities that make hysterectomy an extremely high-risk surgery. However, based on findings from other studies, this patient's age, race, surgical history, obesity, and chronic pain increase her risk of failure with endometrial ablation, and thus hysterectomy is likely the better choice for her. In addition, with her young age and prior tubal ligation, she is at high risk for post ablation tubal sterilization syndrome.

References

1. Dickersin K, Munro MG, Clark M, Langenberg P, Scherer R, Frick K, et al. Surgical Treatment Outcomes Project for Dysfunctional Uterine Bleeding (STOP-DUB) Research Group. Hysterectomy compared with endometrial ablation for dysfunctional uterine bleeding: a randomized controlled trial. *Obstet Gynecol.* 2007;110(6):1279–1289.

2. Dickersin K, Munro M, Langenberg P, Scherer R, Frick KD, Weber AM, et al. Surgical Treatments Outcomes Project for Dysfunctional Uterine Bleeding (STOP DUB): design and methods. *Control Clin Trials.* 2003;591–609.

3. Lethaby A, Shepperd S, Cooke I, Farquhar C. Endometrial resection and ablation versus hysterectomy for heavy menstrual bleeding. *Cochrane Database Syst Rev.* 2000;2.

4. Aberdeen Endometrial Ablation Trials Group. A randomized trial of endometrial ablation versus hysterectomy for the treatment of dysfunctional uterine bleeding: outcome at four years. *Br J Obstet Gynaecol.* 1999;106:360–366.

5. Matteson KA, Abed H, Wheeler TL 2nd, Sung VW, Rahn DD, Schaffer JI, Balk EM, Society of Gynecologic Surgeons Systematic Review Group. A systematic review comparing hysterectomy with less-invasive treatments for abnormal uterine bleeding. *J Minim Invasive Gynecol.* 2012 Jan–Feb;19(1):13–28.

6. Ahonkallio S, Martikainen H, Santala M. Endometrial thermal balloon ablation has a beneficial long-term effect on menorrhagia. *Acta Obstet Gynecol Scand.* 2008;87:107–110.

7. Klebanoff J, Makai GE, Patel NR, Hoffman MK. Incidence and predictors of failed second-generation endometrial ablation. *Gynecol Surg.* 2017;14(1):26.

8. Cramer MS, Klebanoff JS, Hoffman MK. Pain is an independent risk factor for failed global endometrial ablation. *J Minim Invasive Gynecol.* 2018 Sep–Oct;25(6):1018–1023.

9. Smithling KR, Savella G, Raker CA, Matteson KA. Preoperative uterine bleeding pattern and risk of endometrial ablation failure. *Am J Obstet Gynecol.* 2014 Nov;211(5):556.e1–6.

10. American College of Obstetricians and Gynecologists. ACOG Practice Bulletin No. 81: endometrial ablation. *Obstet Gynecol.* 2007(reaffirmed 2018);109:1233–1248.

Pelvic Organ Function After Total Versus Subtotal Abdominal Hysterectomy

SUSAN TSAI, JESSICA TRAYLOR, AND MAGDY MILAD

"Neither total nor subtotal abdominal hysterectomy adversely affects pelvic organ function."

—R. THAKAR ET AL.[1]

Research Question: Does subtotal abdominal hysterectomy result in better pelvic organ function, more rapid rate of recovery, and a reduced rate of complications as compared to total abdominal hysterectomy?

Funding: Grant from the Responsive Funding Programme, Research and Development, National Health Service Executive (SPGS 202)

Study Years: January 1996 to April 2000

Year Study Published: 2002

Study Location: 2 London hospitals

Who Was Studied: Women offered hysterectomy for benign indications

Who Was Excluded: Age >60, suspected cancer, body weight >100 kg, previous pelvic surgery, known endometriosis, abnormal cervical cytology, symptomatic uterine prolapse, symptomatic urinary incontinence

How Many Patients: 279

Study Overview: See Figure 41.1

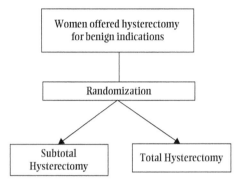

Figure 41.1. Study overview

Study Intervention: Women were randomly assigned to subtotal or total abdominal hysterectomy for benign conditions. Both patients and the investigator who evaluated the outcomes were unaware of treatment assignments for the duration of the study. Each operation was performed with the use of clamp-cut-ligate method, polyglycolic suture, and antibiotic prophylaxis. Electrocoagulation was applied to the endocervical canal during subtotal abdominal hysterectomy. Bilateral salpingo-oophorectomy was performed based on surgeon discretion or patient request.

Follow-Up: 12 months

Endpoints:

- Complications: Intraoperative (e.g., blood loss requiring transfusion) and postoperative (fever, urinary retention, vault hematoma, wound infection, cyclical vaginal bleeding, cervical prolapse, and persistent pelvic pain).
- Urinary and bowel function.
- Sexual function.

RESULTS

- Total abdominal hysterectomy was associated with a significantly longer duration of surgery, greater blood loss, and longer hospital stay. Pre- and

Table 41.1. SUMMARY OF KEY RESULTS

Outcome	Total Hysterectomy (n = 146)	Subtotal Hysterectomy (n = 133)	p-value
Operative time, minutes	71.1 ± 23.4	59.5 ± 20.6	<0.001
Blood loss, mL	422.6 ± 301.8	320.1 ± 271	0.004
Hospital stay, days	6.0± 4.7	5.2 ± 1.1	0.04
Cyclic vaginal bleeding, n	—	9 (6.7)	
Urinary function at	24/121 (19.8)	28/119 (23.5)	0.26
12 months, n/total (%)	1.5 ± 0.9	1.5 ± 0.9	0.74
Urinary frequency			
Stress			
Incontinence[a]			
Bowel function at	18 (14.8)	7 (5.9)	1.00
12 mo, n (%)	43 (35.2)	36 (30.3)	0.20
Constipation			
Urgency			

Data reported as mean ± SD where appropriate.
[a]Data defined as a score on a 4-point scale (1 = never; 2 = occasionally; 3 = weekly; 4 = always).

   postoperative rates of urinary complaints (defined as frequent urination, stress incontinence, urgency, urge incontinence, poor stream, interrupted stream, and incomplete bladder emptying) did not differ between those who underwent total abdominal hysterectomy versus subtotal hysterectomy. See Table 41.1.
- At 6 and 12 months, for those who underwent urodynamic follow-up, there was a reduction in stress incontinence in both groups following surgery.
- No significant differences were found between both groups postoperatively regarding bowel function (rates of constipation, hard stools, urgency, straining, use of laxatives, and incontinence of flatus).
- There was a statistically significant increase in frequency of sexual activity postoperatively in both groups independent on type of surgery.
- At 12 months, 6.8% of women in the subtotal hysterectomy group had cyclical vaginal bleeding.

Criticisms and Limitations:

- The study excluded women with a body weight >100 kg, which limits generalizability to obese patients.
- The route of hysterectomy for all women included in the study was an abdominal approach, which may limit external validity of this study when considering other routes of surgery (e.g., laparoscopic); however, there is a growing body of literature that does not support clinically important differences in complications or outcomes between total versus subtotal laparoscopic hysterectomy.[2]
- The study examined urinary pre- and postoperative urinary function according to the presence or absence of fibroids and found that women with fibroids had a greater reduction in micturition frequency postop. Fibroids have other associated symptoms including dyspareunia and heavy menstrual bleeding that can impact sexual function. A similar subset analysis of the impact of hysterectomy on sexual function in women with and without fibroids could deepen our understanding of the impact of this potential confounder.
- The difference in operative time of 11.6 minutes for total versus subtotal hysterectomy is reported as statistically significant, but the clinical significance of this may vary based on clinical setting (e.g., presence of trainees, operating room turnover times, case volumes). The increased operative time with total abdominal hysterectomy may be offset by the decreased need for Pap smears and elimination of the risk of cyclic bleeding postoperatively.

Other Relevant Studies and Information:

- Another prospective study similarly showed no adverse effects on urinary symptoms when patients were assessed at 12 months postoperatively after abdominal hysterectomy.[3]
- The majority of studies assessing sexual function after hysterectomy have found no adverse effects.[4–8]
- In long-term follow-up of a multicenter, randomized clinical trial, with an average of 14 years since abdominal hysterectomy, more women undergoing subtotal hysterectomy (33%) seemed to have subjective urinary incontinence compared to total abdominal hysterectomy (20%), although this result was not confirmed by multiple imputation analysis. There were also no significant differences in any secondary

outcomes including pelvic organ prolapse, constipation, or satisfaction with sex life.[9]

- A large Cochrane review comparing total versus subtotal hysterectomy showed no evidence of a difference in urinary, bowel, or sexual function between the two procedures.[9] Most of studies included in the review compared abdominal surgeries, but a smaller number of studies did compare total versus subtotal hysterectomies performed laparoscopically.
- American Association of Gynecologic Laparoscopists (AAGL) guidelines state that there is no clear evidence to support supracervical hysterectomy; the decision should be left up to the surgeon and their patient. Care should be taken if morcellation is performed to remove all the uterine tissue.[2]

Summary and Implications: Significant adverse effects on pelvic organ function are not common after subtotal or total abdominal hysterectomy. Based on this and other studies, American Association of Gynecologic Laparoscopists (AAGL)guidelines indicate that both subtotal or total abdominal hysterectomy are appropriate for women with benign uterine disease.

CLINICAL CASE: PELVIC ORGAN FUNCTION AFTER TOTAL VERSUS SUBTOTAL ABDOMINAL HYSTERECTOMY

Case History

A 50-year-old G1P1 with abnormal uterine bleeding and symptomatic fibroids for many years presents for consultation. Following extensive discussion about options for both her bleeding and fibroids, the patient opted to proceed with definitive therapy with a hysterectomy. She had a past history of abnormal pap that required a LEEP for severe dysplasia 5 years ago but asks her gynecologist if she should keep her cervix to preserve sexual function.

Based on the results of the Thakar paper, how should the patient be counseled about which hysterectomy is best for her?

Suggested Answer

The Thakar trial showed that there was no difference in urinary, bowel, and sexual function following hysterectomy; either subtotal or total.

The patient in this scenario should be counseled toward a total hysterectomy. Current evidence does not support the superiority of subtotal hysterectomy in terms of bowel, bladder, or sexual function. Additionally, with her history of dysplasia requiring intervention, she should be counseled that, given her history, performing a subtotal hysterectomy would require continued surveillance for another 20 years, and if her Pap smears were abnormal, requiring colposcopy which showed dysplasia again, that this may require future surgery for trachelectomy.

She should also be counseled about the pros and cons of removing the fallopian tubes and ovaries at the time of hysterectomy.

References

1. Thakar R, Ayers S, Clarkson P, Stanton S, Manyonda I. Outcomes after Total versus subtotal abdominal hysterectomy. *N Engl J Med.* 2002;347 (17):1318–1325. doi:10.1056/NEJMoa013336.
2. American Association of Gynecologic Laparoscopists. AAGL practice report: practice guidelines for laparoscopic subtotal/supracervical hysterectomy (LSH). *J Minim Invasive Gynecol.* 2014;21(1):9–16.
3. Virtanen H, Makinen J, Tenho T, Kiilholma P, Pitkanen Y, Hirvonen T. Effects of abdominal hysterectomy on urinary and sexual symptoms. *Br J Urol.* 1993;72(6):868–872.
4. Rhodes JC, Kjerulff KH, Langenberg PW, Guzinski GM. Hysterectomy and sexual functioning. *JAMA.* 1999;282(20):1934–1941.
5. Helstrom L, Lundberg PO, Sorbom D, Backstrom T. Sexuality after hysterectomy: a factor analysis of women's sexual lives before and after subtotal hysterectomy. *Obstet Gyneco.* 1993;81(3):357–362.
6. Coppen A, Bishop M, Beard RJ, Barnard GJ, Collins WP. Hysterectomy, hormones, and behaviour. A prospective study. *Lancet.* 1981;1(8212):126–128.
7. Doganay M, Kokanali D, Kokanali MK, Cavkaytar S, Aksakal OS. Comparison of female sexual function in women who underwent abdominal or vaginal hysterectomy with or without bilateral salpingo-oophorectomy. *J Gynecol Obstet Hum Reprod.* 2018.
8. Berlit S, Tuschy B, Wuhrer A, et al. Sexual functioning after total versus subtotal laparoscopic hysterectomy. *Arch Gynecol Obstet.* 2018;298(2):337–344.
9. Lethaby A, Mukhopadhyay A, Naik R. Total versus subtotal hysterectomy for benign gynaecological conditions. *Cochrane Database Syst Rev.* 2012(4):CD004993.

Prolonged GnRH Agonist and Add-Back Therapy for Symptomatic Endometriosis

SIERRA J. SEAMAN AND HYE-CHUN HUR

"GnRH agonist [with "add-back" therapy] administered to symptomatic endometriosis patients for 12 months provides extended pain relief and bone mineral density preservation."

— ES Surrey et al.[1]

Research Question: Among women with symptomatic endometriosis who are receiving GnRH agonist therapy, what is the impact of various add-back hormonal therapies versus placebo with respect to pain and bone mineral density?

Funding: Grant support from TAP Pharmaceutical Products, Inc.

Year Study Began: Not specified

Year Study Published: 2002

Study Location: 26 study sites across the United States

Who Was Studied: This was a follow-up study with post-treatment analysis of women with surgically confirmed endometriosis undergoing prolonged Lupron treatment for one year.[2] The original clinical trial included 18- to 43-year-old women with symptomatic endometriosis surgically diagnosed within 12 months of preliminary study enrollment.[2] Women who completed at least 280 days of

Lupron treatment were included in this follow-up study. The follow-up period began 29 days after the last leuprolide acetate injection.

Who Was Excluded: Women who completed fewer than 280 days of treatment with leuprolide acetate. Women with irregular menses.

How Many Patients: 201 (original clinical trial), 123 (follow-up study), 60 (entering the second year of follow-up)

Study Overview: See Figure 42.1

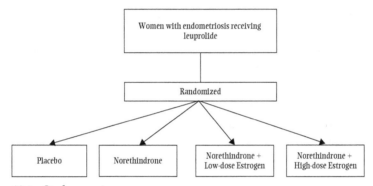

Figure 42.1. Study overview

Study Intervention: In the original study, all patients received monthly leuprolide and were randomized to one of four treatments for 52 weeks: (a) placebo, (b) progestin only, (c) progestin and low-dose estrogen, or (d) progestin and high-dose estrogen. Both patients and providers were blinded to the treatment. This was a follow-up study monitoring post-treatment pelvic pain symptoms and bone mineral density up to 2 years following prolonged 12-month treatment with GnRH-agonist with either placebo or one of three add-back therapies.

Follow-Up: Patients were monitored for 2 years at regular intervals using validated pain scores and physical exam findings. Bone mineral density was monitored every 4 months starting at month 8 until return to baseline.

Endpoints: The primary outcome was change in pain symptoms (dysmenorrhea, nonmenstrual pelvic pain, deep dyspareunia) and pelvic exam findings (tenderness and induration). The secondary outcome was change in bone mineral density.

RESULTS

- 123 of the 201 patients in the original study completed at least 280 days of leuprolide acetate treatment and were enrolled in this follow-up study. Sixty-three of the 123 follow-up patients did not complete the 2-year post-treatment follow-up (50% drop-out rate) due to pregnancy, patient request, worsening symptoms, need for additional therapy, loss to follow-up, noncompliance, or other.
- All groups who received extended leuprolide acetate treatment had comparable improvement in pain symptoms and exam benefits, but groups with add-back therapy had less bone loss.
- All groups who received extended leuprolide acetate treatment had a lengthened time interval to recurrent symptoms with pain scores remaining below baseline for 8+ months after completion of therapy.
- Patients who received high-dose estrogen as part of their add-back therapy had a faster return to menses and dysmenorrhea than the other treatment groups.
- Bone mineral density remained at or above baseline in all add-back groups.
- Bone density loss in the placebo group reversed slowly and did not return to baseline by final follow-up visit. See Table 42.1.

Table 42.1. LONG-TERM OUTCOMES OF EXTENDED 12-MONTH LUPRON TREATMENT

Change in Pelvic Pain Score

	Follow–Up Month 1	Follow–Up Month 4	Follow–Up Month 8	Follow–Up Month 12
Lupron	−2	−1	−1	−1
Lupron + Aygestin	−1	−2	−1	−1
Lupron + Aygestin + Premarin 0.625mg	−1	−1	−1	−1
Lupron + Aygestin + Premarin 1.25mg	−1	−1	−1	−1

Percent Change in Bone Mineral Density Score

	Last Lupron Injection	Follow–Up Month 8	Follow–Up Month 12	Follow–Up Month 24
Lupron	−5.4	−3.4	−2.3	−0.9
Lupron + Aygestin	−1.2	−0.9	−0.7	1.5
Lupron + Aygestin + Premarin 0.625mg	−0.2	0.2	0.8	1.2
Lupron + Aygestin + Premarin 1.25mg	0.5	0.6	0.5	0.9

Criticisms and Limitations: The final sample size for the 24-month study period was quite small due to a 50% drop-out rate during the 2-year post-treatment period. There was no prospective power calculation for the follow-up study. The number of patients with Stage III and Stage IV endometriosis were particularly small; it is unclear whether GnRH agonists used in conjunction with aygestin would result in a similar decrease in pelvic pain for patients with advanced disease.

Other Relevant Studies and Information:

- GnRH agonists have been shown to be effective for managing symptoms of severe endometriosis.[3]
- Use of add-back therapy for treatment of hypoestrogenic side effects resulting with short-term use of GnRH agonists has also been well studied.[4,5]
- Previous studies on long-term effects on bone mineral loss following 6 months of treatment with GnRH agonists alone did not show a return to baseline after 6 to 12 months, also suggesting GnRH agonists should not be administered for prolonged periods of time without appropriate add-back therapy.[5]
- The American College of Obstetricians and Gynecologists recommends that when GnRH agonist is used for endometrial pain relief, add-back therapy should be implemented to reduce GnRH agonist associated bone loss and provide symptomatic relief.[6]

Summary and Implications: Twelve-month extended use of GnRH agonists with and without add-back therapy is effective for the treatment of endometriosis and extends the duration of symptom relief for 8+ months post-treatment. Appropriate add-back therapy is an important treatment adjunct to GnRH agonists for preservation of bone mineral density.

CLINICAL CASE

Case History

A 30-year-old woman with surgically confirmed endometriosis presents to your office with a chief complaint of ongoing pelvic pain and dysmenorrhea. Use of NSAIDS and combined oral contraceptives have failed to relieve her symptoms. She desires a long-term solution for her symptoms. She has heard about GnRH agonists but is worried about side effects including vasomotor symptoms and osteoporosis. How do you counsel this patient?

Suggested Answer

GnRH agonists are highly effective at controlling symptoms of endometriosis. Prior studies have demonstrated that the simultaneous use of add-back therapy controls vasomotor symptoms. In addition, the patient is counseled regarding the importance of daily aygestin treatment for preservation of bone mineral density. This study suggests extended use of GnRH agonists with appropriate add-back therapy not only prolongs symptom control through the 12-month treatment period but also offers an additional 8+ months of symptom control after completion of treatment. For reproductive-aged patients who wish to conceive, conservative surgical treatment for endometriosis-related pelvic pain with laparoscopic excision or fulguration of endometriosis may be a better option. All treatment options for endometriosis should be thoroughly discussed with the patient, and the plan of care should be tailored to the patient's medical profile, age, and reproductive goals.

References

1. Surrey ES, Hornstein MD. Add-Back Study Group. Prolonged GnRH agonist and add-back therapy for symptomatic endometriosis: long-term follow-up. *Obstet Gynecol.* 2002;99(5):709–719.
2. Hornstein MD, Surrey ES, Weisberg GW, Casino LA. Lupron Add-Back Study Group. Leuprolide acetate depot and hormonal add-back in endometriosis: a 12-month study. *Obstet Gynecol.* 1998;91:16–24.
3. Dlugi AM, Miller JD, Knittle J. Lupron Study Group. Lupron Depot (leuprolide acetate for depot suspension) in the treatment of endometriosis: a randomized, placebo-controlled, double-blind study. *Fertil Steril.* 1990;54:419–427.
4. Gargiulo AR, Hornstein MD. The role of GnRH agonists plus add-back therapy in the treatment of endometriosis. *Sem Reprod Endocrinol.* 1997;15:3.
5. Surrey ES. Add-back therapy and gonadotropin-releasing hormone agonists in the treatment of patients with endometriosis: can a consensus be reached? *Fertil Steril.* 1999;71(3):420–424.
6. Management of endometriosis. Practice Bulletin No. 114. American College of Obstetricians and Gynecologists. *Obstet Gynecol.* 2010;116:223–236.

Laparoscopic Excision Versus Ablation for Endometriosis-Associated Pain

LAURA NEWCOMB AND NICOLE DONNELLAN

"The limited available evidence demonstrates that at 12 months post-surgery, symptoms of dysmenorrhea, dyschezia, and chronic pelvic pain secondary to endometriosis are significantly improved with laparoscopic excision compared with ablation surgery."

—J PUNDIR ET AL.[1]

Research Question: Should patients with endometriosis-associated pain who desire surgical intervention undergo laparoscopic excision or ablation of endometriosis?

Funding: Not disclosed

Year Study Began: One study began in 2001, one in 2002, and the third did not disclose study dates

Year Study Published: 2017

Study Location: The trials were conducted in the United Kingdom and Australia.

Who Was Studied: Women ages 18 or older with endometriosis-associated pain and surgically diagnosed endometriosis. One study included only women with stage 1 disease according to the revised American Society for Reproductive Medicine guidelines, and 2 studies included women with stage 1-3 disease.

Who Was Excluded: Women concurrently using hormonal therapy, pregnant, or breastfeeding. Women with advanced stage 4 disease were also excluded.

How Many Patients: 198

Study Overview: See Figure 43.1

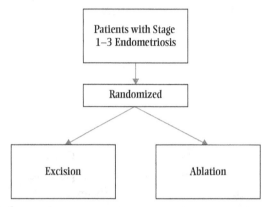

Figure 43.1. Study overview

Study Intervention: Participants in the trials were randomized to undergo either laparoscopic excision using either monopolor scissors or harmonic scalpel or laparoscopic ablation of endometriotic implants by monopolar laparoscopic scissors or CO2 laser vaporization.

Follow-Up: Up to 6 months in 1 study and 12 months in the other 2 studies

Endpoints: Primary outcome: Difference in preoperative and postoperative visual analog scores (VAS) scores for dysmenorrhea. Secondary outcomes: Reduction in VAS scores for dyspareunia, dyschezia, and chronic pelvic pain.

RESULTS

- Three randomized control trials were included in this meta-analysis.[2-4]
- The excision group had a greater reduction in VAS scores for dysmenorrhea compared with ablation ($p = 0.05$). See Table 43.1.

- Pooling results of 2 of the included studies, the excision group had a significantly greater reduction in VAS scores for dyspareunia compared with ablation ($p = 0.07$).
- Pooling results of 2 of the included studies, the excision group had a significantly greater reduction in VAS scores for dyschezia compared with ablation ($p = 0.009$).
- One study evaluated chronic pelvic pain; excision resulted in a greater reduction in chronic pelvic pain compared with ablation ($p < 0.01$).
- One study evaluated reduction in pelvic pain; there was no significant difference with excision or ablation ($p = 0.87$).
- One study reported on the Endometriosis Health Profile (EHP-30) core pain score; this study showed that excision resulted in a greater reduction in EHP-30 than ablation ($p = 0.001$).

Table 43.1. MEAN DIFFERENCE IN VAS SCORES FOR PRIMARY AND SECONDARY OUTCOMES

	Excision (n)	Ablation (n)	Mean Difference in VAS Scores (MD [95% CI], *p*-value)
Primary Outcome			
Dysmenorrhea	10	96	0.99 [−0.02–2.00] $p = 0.05$
Secondary Outcomes			
Dyspareunia	102	96	0.96 [−0.07–1.99] $p = 0.07$
Dyschezia	102	96	1.31 [0.33–2.29] $p = 0.009$
Chronic Pelvic Pain	48	47	2.57 [1.27–3.87] $p = 0.0001$

Abbreviations: VAS, visual analog scale; CI, confidence interval.

Criticisms and Limitations: Only 2 studies were eligible for inclusion in this meta-analysis, underscoring the need for further well-designed research studies in this area. Some limitations in analysis exist in the studies included in the meta-analysis—the Healey group[3] did not describe in detail any possible variations between excision techniques, for example. Further, this study included patients with stages 1–3 of disease as one group; a difference may exist in treatment efficacy between different groups. Last, there are other co-existing diagnoses that could contribute to pelvic pain (including adenomyosis, gastrointestinal, genitourinary, and musculoskeletal disorders) that were not accounted for.

Other Relevant Studies and Information:

- The only other existing meta-analysis on this topic was performed by the Cochrane group[5] and published in 2014. Evidence for the reduction of pain at 12 months was based only on the results of 1 study (the Healey et al. study). That review concluded that ablation and excision were associated with a reduction in pain and that excision leads to a reduction in pain at 6 and 12 months when compared with diagnostic laparoscopy.
- The Healey group has subsequently performed a 5-year follow-up study on the same cohort of patients included in this article. Symptom reduction persisted through this time frame, and excision was persistently more effective than ablation for treatment of dyspareunia 5 years following surgery.[6]
- The American College of Obstetricians and Gynecologists endorses conservative surgical management as an option for pain relief in patients with endometriosis but does caution that there is a high rate of recurrence.[7]

Summary and Implications: This systematic review and meta-analysis concludes that at 12 months post-surgery, symptoms of dysmenorrhea, dyschezia, and chronic pelvic pain secondary to endometriosis showed a significantly greater improvement with laparoscopic excision compared with ablation. Based on the data reported in this analysis, excision of endometriosis is recommended for women with stages 1–3 endometriosis.

CLINICAL CASE

Case History

A 29-year-old G0 with a history of a prior diagnostic laparoscopy with surgically diagnosed stage 2 endometriosis was placed on hormonal contraception for several years. She initially complained of only cyclic dysmenorrhea, but her pain is now more severe and occurring outside of her menses. She misses a few days of work each month due to pain. She had a recent normal appearing ultrasound without evidence of endometrioma. You are her surgeon and she now desires surgical intervention for pain relief. Should you perform laparoscopic excision or ablation of her endometriosis?

Suggested Answer

This patient is a good surgical candidate based on her history and current symptoms. While the patient must be counseled that surgery comes with more risks than medical or conservative management, surgery is warranted in her case given that she has pain that is interfering with her life activities and she has attempted and failed hormonal management. Based on the most up-to-date literature, this systematic review and meta-analysis suggests that excision is the superior method of surgical treatment for her endometriosis. The patient in this vignette is typical of patients who were included in the review, thus she should be treated with excision of endometriosis following attempts at medical/hormonal management. Other forms of hormonal management could be considered based on her risk factors if she prefers not to undergo surgery.

References

1. Pundir J, Omanwa K, Kovoor E, Pundir V, Lancaster G, Barton-Smith P. Laparoscopic excision versus ablation for endometriosis-associated pain: an updated systematic review and meta-analysis. *J Minim Invasive Gynecol*. 2017;24(5):747–756. doi:10.1016/j.jmig.2017.04.008
2. PBS. An investigation of the surgical treatment of endometriosis. 2010. http://ethos.bl.uk.
3. Healey M, Ang WC, Cheng C. Surgical treatment of endometriosis: a prospective randomized double-blinded trial comparing excision and ablation. *Fertil Steril*. 2010;94(7):2536–2540. doi:10.1016/j.fertnstert.2010.02.044
4. Wright J, Lotfallah H, Jones K, Lovell D. A randomized trial of excision versus ablation for mild endometriosis. *Fertil Steril*. 2005;83(6):1830–1836. doi:10.1016/j.fertnstert.2004.11.066
5. Duffy JMN, Arambage K, Correa FJS, et al. Laparoscopic surgery for endometriosis. *Cochrane Database Syst Rev*. 2014;4:CD011031. doi:10.1002/14651858.CD011031.pub2
6. Healey M, Cheng C, Kaur H. To excise or ablate endometriosis? A prospective randomized double-blinded trial after 5-year follow-up. *J Minim Invasive Gynecol*. 2014;21(6):999–1004. doi:10.1016/j.jmig.2014.04.002
7. Practice Bulletin No. 114: management of endometriosis. *Obstet Gynecol*. 2010 Jul;116(1):223–236. doi:10.1097/AOG.0b013e3181e8b073. PubMed PMID: 20567196

44

Clomiphene, Metformin, or Both for Infertility With Polycystic Ovarian Syndrome

The PPCOS Trial

TANA KIM AND ZARAQ KHAN

"[This] study supports the use of clomiphene citrate alone as first-line therapy for infertility in women with the polycystic ovary syndrome."
— RS LEGRO ET AL.[1]

Research Question: Should infertile women with polycystic ovarian syndrome (PCOS) receive clomiphene, metformin, or both for ovulation induction?

Funding: National Institutes of Health/National Institute of Child Health and Human Development

Year Study Began: 2002

Year Study Published: 2007

Study Location: 12 centers in the United States

Who Was Studied: Infertile women aged 18 to 39 years with diagnosis of PCOS based on hyperandrogenemia (elevated testosterone level within previous year) and oligomenorrhea (no more than 8 spontaneous menses per year).

Who Was Excluded: Women with other causes of infertility such as abnormal uterine cavity, blocked fallopian tubes, abnormal semen analysis, and women with other causes of amenorrhea like hyperprolactinemia, thyroid disease, congenital adrenal hyperplasia, or clinical suspicion of Cushing's syndrome or androgen secreting neoplasms.

How Many Patients: 626

Study Overview: See Figure 44.1

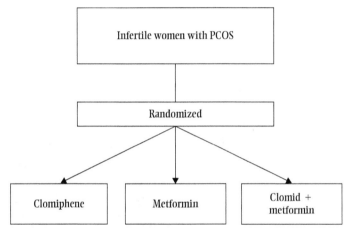

Figure 44.1. Study overview: the PPCOS Trial

Live birth rates among infertile women with PCOS were compared between those who received clomiphene, metformin, or both.

Study Intervention: Women were assigned to 3 treatment arms in a double-blind, randomized fashion. The 3 arms included clomiphene plus placebo, extended-release metformin plus placebo, and clomiphene plus extended-release metformin. Women randomized to metformin started with 1 pill once a day (extended-release metformin 500mg or placebo) and titrated up to 2 pills twice a day. Women randomized to clomiphene started with 1 pill once a day (clomiphene 50mg days 3 to 7 of each cycle) and titrated up to 3 pills once a day depending on ovulatory response. Women were treated up to 6 cycles. All study medications were discontinued with a positive pregnancy test. The study was designed as an intention to treat analysis.

Follow-Up: Women were followed until ultrasound confirmation of pregnancy and subsequent obstetrical records and birth outcomes were collected.

Endpoints: Primary outcome: Live birth rate. Secondary outcomes: Rate of ovulation, conception, pregnancy loss, multiple gestation pregnancies, and serious adverse events.

RESULTS

- The clomiphene plus metformin arm had a higher rate of ovulation compared to clomiphene or metformin only arms, but there was no significant difference in live birth rate between clomiphene plus metformin and clomiphene alone. See Table 44.1.
- The live birth rate was 22.5% in the clomiphene arm, 7.2% in the metformin arm, and 26.8% in the clomiphene plus metformin arm.
- The relationship between treatment and live birth was similar in post hoc analyses of subgroups stratified according to body mass index (BMI) ($<30 \, kg/m^2$, 30 to 34 kg/m^2, and $\geq 35 \, kg/m^2$) and whether or not patients had prior fertility treatments.
- The rate of ovulation was highest in the clomiphene plus metformin group at 60.4% while the ovulation rate was 49% in the clomiphene only and 29% in the metformin only arms.
- There was no difference in total pregnancy loss between the 3 arms.
- The rate of multiple gestation pregnancy was 6.0% with clomiphene, 0% with metformin, and 3.1% with clomiphene and metformin. This difference was not statistically significant.

Table 44.1. COMPARISON OF PREGNANCY OUTCOMES IN WOMEN
ON CLOMIPHENE, METFORMIN, OR CLOMIPHENE AND METFORMIN
FOR OVULATION INDUCTION

Outcomes (%)	Clomiphene % ($n = 209$)	Metformin % ($n = 208$)	Both % ($n = 209$)	p-value B vs. M	p-value B vs. C	p-value C vs. M
Ovulation	49.0	29.0	60.4	<0.001	0.003	<0.001
Conception	29.7	12.0	38.3	<0.001	0.06	<0.001
Pregnancy loss	25.8	40.0	30.0	0.35	0.58	0.19
Pregnancy	23.9	8.7	31.1	<0.001	0.10	<0.001
Singleton	94.0	100	96.9	0.96	0.45	0.95
Twins	4.0	0	3.1	1.0	1.0	1.0
Triplets	2.0	0	0	1.0	1.0	1.0
Live birth	22.5	7.2	26.8	<0.001	0.31	<0.001

Abbreviations: C, clomiphene; M, metformin; B, both.

- Serious adverse events, primarily related to pregnancy, were more common in the clomiphene (3.3%) and clomiphene plus metformin (5.3%) groups than among the metformin only (1.0%) group.

Criticisms and Limitations: Routine ultrasound monitoring of follicular development and endometrial response were not included in the protocol. All women had timed intercourse and were not permitted to trigger ovulation with human chorionic gonadotropin or utilize intrauterine insemination. All women received extended-release metformin due to its increased tolerability; however, extended release may be less efficacious than the immediate-release formulation in women with PCOS. As metformin was discontinued at the time of positive pregnancy test, continued effects of metformin throughout early pregnancy remained unknown. Additionally, the study was not adequately powered to detect a difference in the pregnancy loss rate among the 3 arms.

Other Relevant Studies and Information:

- Other randomized clinical trials assessing live birth outcomes have also demonstrated no additional benefit in adding metformin to clomiphene for ovulation induction in women with PCOS.[2,3]
- Although previous studies have demonstrated effectiveness of metformin on ovulation and pregnancy rates, live birth rates were not studied as an outcome.[4–7]
- Newer data from the PPCOS II trial now supports the use of aromatase inhibitors like letrozole over clomiphene as first-line therapy for treatment of infertility in women with PCOS.[8]

Summary and Implications: In women with infertility due to PCOS-related anovulation, clomiphene monotherapy resulted in greater live birth rates than metformin monotherapy. Using metformin in conjunction with clomiphene did not significantly improve live birth rates compared to clomiphene alone. These findings support the use of clomiphene monotherapy for women experiencing PCOS-related infertility.

CLINICAL CASE: CLOMIPHENE, METFORMIN, OR BOTH FOR INFERTILITY WITH PCOS

Case History

A 28-year-old nulliparous woman with irregular periods and hirsutism presents to your office for infertility. Her menstrual history is notable for unpredictable periods occurring approximately 8 times per year. Additionally, she complains of increased hair growth on her face and abdomen. Serum testosterone level comes back slightly elevated, but all other labs are normal. A fertility workup demonstrates normal uterus with patent fallopian tubes and a normal semen analysis. Based on the PPCOS trial, what medication should you offer this patient for ovulation induction and how would you counsel her regarding side effects?

Suggested Answer

Based on this patient's clinical history of irregular menstrual cycles and hyperandrogenism, she likely has PCOS. With patent fallopian tubes, ovulation induction is an option for fertility treatment. The PPCOS trial concluded that there was no benefit of combination therapy with clomiphene plus metformin in terms of live birth rates in women with PCOS. Therefore, first-line therapy for ovulation induction based on the PPCOS trial should be clomiphene alone. However, newer data from a subsequent study, the PPCOS II trial, demonstrated higher cumulative ovulation and live birth rates with letrozole compared to clomiphene (61.7% vs. 48.3% for ovulation and 27.5% vs. 19.1% for live birth) in women with PCOS. Therefore, letrozole is now the recommended first-line ovulation induction agent for women with PCOS. For women with non-PCOS related infertility, such as unexplained infertility, clomiphene is still considered an appropriate option for ovulation induction. Side effects of clomiphene include risk of multiple gestation, hot flashes, and, rarely, visual disturbances. Side effects of letrozole include risk of multiple gestation, hot flashes, fatigue, and dizziness.

References

1. Legro RS, et al. Clomiphene, metformin, or both for infertility in the polycystic ovary syndrome. *N Engl J Med.* 2007;356(6):551–566.
2. Moll E, et al. Effect of clomifene citrate plus metformin and clomifene citrate plus placebo on induction of ovulation in women with newly diagnosed polycystic ovary syndrome: randomised double blind clinical trial. *BMJ.* 2006;332(7556):1485.

3. Zain MM, et al. Comparison of clomiphene citrate, metformin, or the combination of both for first-line ovulation induction, achievement of pregnancy, and live birth in Asian women with polycystic ovary syndrome: a randomized controlled trial. *Fertil Steril.* 2009;91(2):514–521.

4. Lord JM, Flight IH, Norman RJ. Metformin in polycystic ovary syndrome: systematic review and meta-analysis. *BMJ.* 2003;327(7421):951–953.

5. Nestler JE, et al. Effects of metformin on spontaneous and clomiphene-induced ovulation in the polycystic ovary syndrome. *N Engl J Med.* 1998;338(26):1876–1880.

6. Vandermolen DT, et al. Metformin increases the ovulatory rate and pregnancy rate from clomiphene citrate in patients with polycystic ovary syndrome who are resistant to clomiphene citrate alone. *Fertil Steril.* 2001;75(2):310–315.

7. Palomba S, et al. Prospective parallel randomized, double-blind, double-dummy controlled clinical trial comparing clomiphene citrate and metformin as the first-line treatment for ovulation induction in nonobese anovulatory women with polycystic ovary syndrome. *J Clin Endocrinol Metab.* 2005;90(7):4068–4074.

8. Legro RS, et al. Letrozole versus clomiphene for infertility in the polycystic ovary syndrome. *N Engl J Med.* 2014 Jul 10;371(2):119–129.

45

A Randomized Clinical Trial to Evaluate Optimal Treatment for Unexplained Infertility

The FASTT Trial

STEPHANIE ROTHENBERG AND JOSEPH SANFILIPPO

"In this large randomized controlled trial that compared a conventional treatment paradigm to an accelerated strategy to IVF for infertile couples, it was found that gonadotropin/IUI use was of no added value."
—RH REINDOLLAR ET AL.[1]

Research Question: Do couples with unexplained infertility benefit from an accelerated treatment approach, which omits treatment with injectable gonadotropins and intrauterine insemination (IUI)?

Funding: National Institute of Child Health and Human Development

Year Study Began: 2001

Year Study Published: 2010

Study Location: An academic medical center associated with a private infertility center in the United States

Who Was Studied: Couples with unexplained infertility in which the female partner was 21 to 39 years old

Who Was Excluded: Patients not eligible for ovulation induction with IUI, presence of hydrosalpinges, stage III or IV endometriosis, use of donor sperm, need for assisted reproductive technology procedures other than in vitro fertilization (IVF)

How Many Patients: 503 couples

Study Overview: See Figure 45.1

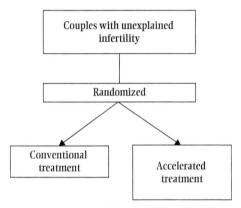

Figure 45.1. Study overview: the FASST Trial

Study Intervention: All couples underwent treatment with clomiphene citrate (CC) and IUI for up to 3 cycles. If they did not conceive, the couples were randomized to either the Conventional Treatment group or the Accelerated Treatment group. Those assigned to the Conventional Treatment arm underwent up to 3 additional treatment cycles with injectable gonadotropins and IUI. If they did not conceive, they then underwent up to 6 cycles of IVF. Those assigned to the Accelerated Treatment arm proceeded immediately with up to 6 cycles of IVF. All treatment protocols were standardized.

Follow-Up: Discharge from the hospital of both mother and baby *or* until 1 year after completing the treatment protocol

Endpoints: Primary outcomes: Time to pregnancy resulting in a live birth and cost per delivery (the ratio of total cost by the number of couples delivering a live-born baby). Secondary outcomes: Per cycle pregnancy rates, per couple pregnancy rates, and adverse events for each treatment. Pregnancy rate was defined as a pregnancy resulting in a live birth or an ongoing pregnancy >20 weeks at the time of study conclusion.

RESULTS

- Patients randomized to the Accelerated Treatment arm had a significantly shorter time to pregnancy resulting in a live birth compared to those in the Conventional Treatment arm (8 months vs. 11 months). See Table 45.1.
- Average charges per delivery were $9,846 lower in the Accelerated Treatment arm. See Table 45.1.
- Per cycle pregnancy rate (defined as live births or ongoing pregnancies >20 weeks) by treatment type was found to be 7.6%, 9.8%, and 30.7% for CC/IUI, gonadotropin/IUI, and IVF, respectively.
- Per couple pregnancy rates were similar between groups at the end of each treatment arm (Conventional Treatment 74.9% vs. Accelerated Treatment 77.7%).

Table 45.1. SUMMARY OF FASTT's KEY FINDINGS

	Conventional Treatment	Accelerated Treatment	*p*-value
Median time to pregnancy resulting in a live birth	11 months	8 months	0.045
Cost per delivery	$71,400	$61,700	0.084

Criticisms and Limitations: Data collection was concluded while 63 couples had an ongoing viable pregnancy but were included to calculate both the per cycle pregnancy rate and the per couple pregnancy rate. The rate of multiple births in couples treated with gonadotropin/IUI was also lower than rates noted in other multicenter randomized trials, which may have been due to standardization of treatment that could be achieved within a single clinical center.[2–5]

The study was performed in a state with mandated insurance coverage for infertility care, which may limit its generalizability. Additionally, insurance charges were used as a surrogate for economic cost during cost-effectiveness comparisons, so caution should be used when looking at absolute value of costs. While suggestive of cost savings for patients in the Accelerated Treatment arm, statistical significance was not reached.

Other Relevant Studies and Information:

- Subsequent randomized clinical trials have supported the findings of FASTT. The Forty and Over Treatment Trial (FORT-T) specifically evaluated the optimal treatment of unexplained infertility in couples with a female partner aged 38 to 42 years. They compared treatment with 2 cycles of ovulation induction (either CC or gonadotropins) and IUI followed by IVF versus proceeding immediately with IVF. They found that the clinical pregnancy rate in couples who commenced IVF immediately underwent 36% fewer treatment cycles and conceived a pregnancy leading to live birth 3.5 months faster.[6] The complementary findings of FASTT and FORT-T have resulted in a significant decline in the use of gonadotropins for ovulation induction for the treatment of unexplained infertility.
- Other studies have found that 3 cycles of gonadotropins and IUI are equivalent in efficacy to IVF in terms of live birth rates, supporting the findings of the FASTT trial.[7]
- Based on the FASTT trial results, the American Society for Reproductive Medicine (ASRM) recommends that couples with unexplained fertility transition to IVF after unsuccessful ovarian stimulation and IUI treatments with oral agents.[8]

Summary and Implications: Couples with unexplained infertility who pursued an accelerated treatment strategy involving immediate IVF therapy following an initial 3 cycles of injectable gonadotropins and IUI had a decreased time to pregnancy compared to those treated with extended cycles of injectable gonadotropins and IUI before proceeding with IVF. The accelerated treatment approach was also less costly per live birth.

CLINICAL CASE

Case History

A 36-year-old female and her 42-year-old male partner presented for fertility evaluation. The patient has regular menses every 30 days, and they have been attempting pregnancy for 15 months with well-timed intercourse. They underwent a complete fertility evaluation, which was unremarkable. Ultimately, they were diagnosed with unexplained infertility. Based on the results of FASTT, what treatment course would you recommend?

Suggested Answer

According to the results of FASTT, the couple would be equally likely to have a live born child with both a conventional treatment approach and an accelerated approach. However, the couple would have a shorter time to pregnancy if treatment with gonadotropins and IUI was omitted. It may also be more cost effective to proceed immediately to IVF if they do not conceive after three cycles of clomiphene and IUI.

References

1. Reindollar RH, Regan MM, Neumann PJ, et al. A randomized clinical trial to evaluate optimal treatment for unexplained infertility: the Fast Track and Standard Treatment (FASTT) trial. *Fertil Steril.* 2010;94:888–899.
2. Guzick DS, Carson SA, Coutifaris C, et al. Efficacy of superovulation and intrauterine insemination in the treatment of infertility. National Cooperative Reproductive Medicine Network. *N Engl J Med.* 1999;340:177–183.
3. Gleicher N, Oleske DM, Tur-Kaspa I, Vidali A, Karande V. Reducing the risk of high-order multiple pregnancy after ovarian stimulation with gonadotropins. *N Engl J Med.* 2000;343:2–7.
4. Dickey RP, Taylor SN, Lu PY, Sartor BM, Rye PH, Pyrzak R. Relationship of follicle numbers and estradiol levels to multiple implantation in 3,608 intrauterine insemination cycles. *Fertil Steril.* 2001;75:69–78.
5. Diamond MP, Legro RS, Coutifaris C, et al. Letrozole, gonadotropin, or clomiphene for unexplained infertility. *N Engl J Med.* 2015;373:1230–1240.
6. Goldman MB, Thornton KL, Ryley D, et al. A randomized clinical trial to determine optimal infertility treatment in older couples: the Forty and Over Treatment Trial (FORT-T). *Fertil Steril.* 2014;101:1574–1581.
7. Nandi A, Bhide P, Hooper R, et al. Intrauterine insemination with gonadotropin stimulation or in vitro fertilization for the treatment of unexplained subfertility: a randomized controlled trial. *Fertil Steril.* 2017;107:1329–1335.
8. Practice Committee of the American Society for Reproductive Medicine. Electronic address: asrm@asrm.org; Practice Committee of the American Society for Reproductive Medicine. Evidence-based treatments for couples with unexplained infertility: a guideline. *Fertil Steril.* 2020;113(2):305–322. doi:10.1016/j.fertnst ert.2019.10.014

46

Reproductive Technologies and the Risk of Birth Defects

CAITLIN SACHA AND JOHN PETROZZA

"Although the large majority of births resulting from assisted conception were free of birth defects, treatment with assisted reproductive technology was associated with an increased risk of birth defects, including cerebral palsy, as compared with spontaneous conception. In the case of ICSI, but not IVF, the increased risk of birth defects persisted after adjustment for maternal age and several other risk factors."

—MJ DAVIES ET AL.[1]

Research Question: Is the increased risk of birth defects observed with assisted reproductive technology (ART) due to the treatment procedures or underlying patient characteristics related to infertility?

Funding: National Health and Medical Research Council and the Australian Research Council

Year Study Began: 1986

Year Study Published: 2012

Study Location: South Australia

Who Was Studied: All women with pregnancies delivered or terminated at or over 20 weeks' gestation, as well as those who underwent terminations at less than 20 weeks' gestation for major birth defects

Who Was Excluded: Mothers younger than 20 years of age and cases of acquired (onset after the perinatal period) cerebral palsy

How Many Patients: 308,974

Study Overview: See Figure 46.1

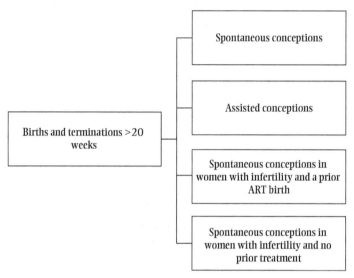

Figure 46.1. Study overview

Study Intervention: Data regarding live births, stillbirths, and terminations at or over 20 weeks' gestation, as well as the use of ART were obtained from the South Australian Perinatal Statistics Collection. Infertility treatment information was obtained from all patients seen at 2 South Australian clinics between 1986 and 2002. Cases of birth defects including major structural, biochemical, or chromosomal defects reported before a child's fifth birthday (including terminations prior to 20 weeks' gestation for birth defects) were identified using the South Australia Birth Defects Register. Minor defects are excluded unless they require treatment or surgical repair.

The authors linked birth outcomes, infertility treatment records, and birth defect data using patient identifiers, unique birth accession numbers, and probabilistic matching software. Factors that could be associated with an increased likelihood of birth defects were controlled in the authors' analyses: maternal age, parity, fetal sex, year of birth, maternal race or ethnicity, maternal nationality, maternal medical comorbidities in pregnancy, maternal smoking during pregnancy, postal code as a proxy for socioeconomic status, and parental occupations. Analyses of singleton and multiple gestation subgroups were performed. The authors did not control for multiple gestation.

Follow-Up: Birth defects were identified through the child's fifth birthday

Endpoints: Prevalence of birth defects

RESULTS

- Assisted conceptions were more likely to be from older, nulliparous, and White women from higher socioeconomic zip codes.
- Of 6163 assisted conceptions, 513 (8.3%) were affected by birth defects, compared to 17,546 (5.8%) of 302,811 spontaneous conceptions in fertile women (adjusted odds ratio [OR] 1.28, 95% confidence interval [CI] 1.16–1.41). Singleton but not multiple gestations were associated with an increased risk of birth defects after assisted conception (Table 46.1). Cardiovascular, musculoskeletal, urogenital, and gastrointestinal defects, as well as cerebral palsy, were more likely to occur in the assisted conception group.
- Intracytoplasmic sperm injection (ICSI) with fresh embryo transfer remained associated with a significantly increased risk of birth defects in singleton pregnancies in adjusted models (Table 46.1). Gamete intrafallopian transfer (GIFT), intrauterine insemination (IUI), and

Table 46.1. SUMMARY OF STUDY FINDINGS FOR COMMONLY USED ART
TREATMENTS

Type of ART	Adjusted OR[a] for Any Birth Defect		All Births (95% CI)
	Singleton Gestations (95%CI)	Multiple Gestations (95% CI)	
Any	1.28 (1.14–1.43)	1.17 (0.91–1.50)	1.26 (1.14–1.40)
IUI	1.46 (1.09–1.95)	0.77 (0.39–1.53)	1.32 (1.01–1.73)
IVF	1.06 (0.87–1.30)	0.99 (0.71–1.37)	1.07 (0.90–1.26)
Fresh transfer	1.05 (0.82–1.35)	1.05 (0.74–1.50)	1.09 (0.89–1.33)
Frozen transfer	1.08 (0.76–1.53)	0.79 (0.39–1.59)	1.02 (0.75–1.39)
ICSI	1.55 (1.24–1.94)	1.39 (0.96–2.01)	1.57 (1.30–1.90)
Fresh transfer	1.73 (1.35–2.21)	1.35 (0.90–2.02)	1.66 (1.35–2.04)
Frozen transfer	1.10 (0.65–1.85)	1.60 (0.71–3.58)	1.28 (0.83–1.99)

[a]OR > 1.0 indicates a higher risk of birth defects in assisted pregnancies compared to spontaneous pregnancies in fertile women.
Abbreviations: OR, odds ratio; ART, assisted reproductive technology; IUI, intrauterine insemination; IVF, in vitro fertilization; ICSI, intracytoplasmic sperm injection.

clomiphene citrate at home also remained associated with an increased risk, though the latter group was quite small.
• Spontaneous conceptions in women with a history of infertility were also associated with an increased risk of birth defects compared to those in fertile women (infertile women with a prior ART pregnancy, adjusted OR 1.25, 95% CI 1.01–1.56; infertile women with no prior treatment, adjusted OR 1.29, 95% CI 0.99–1.68).

Criticisms and Limitations: This study is limited by its retrospective design, as well as its reliance on third-party documentation of birth outcomes and birth defects, which is presumably not blinded to the mode of conception. Importantly, the patient cohort studied was primarily Caucasian, which makes the data less generalizable to more diverse patient populations. Although the authors control for multiple maternal demographic and clinical characteristics, factors associated with a higher risk of birth defects, such as maternal obesity, infertility diagnosis, family history of birth defects, and zygosity of twins, were not available for analysis. In particular, the absence of infertility diagnosis and the limited analysis of spontaneous conceptions in women with a history of infertility reduced the authors' ability to effectively address their primary research question. The demographic characteristics and stimulation protocols for patients undergoing each type of ART are not available, making it difficult to assess the populations undergoing each treatment. Finally, the authors suggest that frozen transfer after ICSI may remove compromised embryos that do not survive thawing; however, if this accounted for the reduced risk of birth defects compared to ICSI fresh transfers, we might expect a reduced risk in in vitro fertilization (IVF) frozen versus fresh transfers, which was not apparent from the data presented.

Other Relevant Studies and Information:

• This study by Davies et al. and several others have supported a small increase in the risk of birth defects in infants conceived with ART, although this risk could be decreasing with time.[1–5]
• Other studies have suggested no increased risk of birth defects with the use of ART. A retrospective cohort study comparing ART and spontaneous pregnancies in infertile women, taking infertility diagnosis into account, failed to show a link between ART and birth defects.[6] Studies assessing whether the rate of birth defects differs by timing of embryo transfer (cleavage vs. blastocyst stage), use of testicular or epididymal sperm compared to conventional IVF and ICSI, or fresh versus frozen embryo transfer have shown no differences.[7–10]

- Based on the available evidence, an American College of Obstetricians and Gynecologists Committee Opinion notes that all patients considering ART should be fully counseled on the potential increased risk of birth defects and, once pregnant, offered routine prenatal ultrasonographic screening for structural anomalies.[11]

Summary and Implications: This study by Davies et al. suggests that the risk of birth defects is modestly increased in assisted conceptions compared to spontaneous conceptions, primarily for singleton gestations and with the use of ICSI with fresh embryo transfer. Infertility diagnosis itself may also be associated with an increased risk of birth defects.

CLINICAL CASE: ART AND THE RISK OF BIRTH DEFECTS

Case History

A 28-year-old otherwise healthy woman and her male partner have been attempting pregnancy for 14 months. A full workup reveals bilaterally obstructed fallopian tubes with otherwise normal testing for both partners. You recommend conventional IVF for treatment. The couple states that they are considering elective ICSI to optimize fertilization and inquire about the risk of birth defects with IVF and ICSI compared to spontaneous conceptions. How would you counsel this couple?

Suggested Answer

This large cohort study demonstrates that once maternal demographic characteristics are controlled, ICSI with fresh embryo transfer seems to have the greatest increased risk of birth defects, including cerebral palsy, compared to spontaneous conceptions in fertile women (adjusted OR 1.73). Based on this data, you might counsel the couple that given normal semen parameters, a more invasive procedure that may carry greater risk would not be your initial recommendation. However, spontaneous conceptions in women with infertility are also associated with an elevated risk of birth defects in this study, and a statistically significant difference in birth defects with a particular intervention may not be clinically significant to a given couple. Ultimately, the couple must weigh the potential risks and benefits of ART intervention with their personal risk threshold and cycle goals.

References

1. Davies MJ, Moore VM, Willson KJ, et al. Reproductive technologies and the risk of birth defects. *N Engl J Med.* 2012;366(19):1803–1813.

2. Hansen M, Kurinczuk JJ, Bower C, Webb S. The risk of major birth defects after intracytoplasmic sperm injection and in vitro fertilization. *N Engl J Med.* 2002;346(10):725–730.

3. Hansen M, Kurinczuk JJ, de Klerk N, Burton P, Bower C. Assisted reproductive technology and major birth defects in Western Australia. *Obstet Gynecol.* 2012;120(4):852–863.

4. Hansen M, Kurinczuk JJ, Milne E, de Klerk N, Bower C. Assisted reproductive technology and birth defects: a systematic review and meta-analysis. *Hum Reprod Update.* 2013;19(4):330–353.

5. Boulet SL, Kirby RS, Reefhuis J, et al. Assisted reproductive technology and birth defects among liveborn infants in Florida, Massachusetts, and Michigan, 2000–2010. *JAMA Pediatr.* 2016;170(6):e154934.

6. Han Y, Luo H, Zhang Y. Congenital anomalies in infants conceived by infertile women through assisted reproductive technology: a cohort study 2004–2014. *Exp Ther Med.* 2018;16:3179–3185.

7. Dar S, Lazer T, Shah PS, Librach CL. Neonatal outcomes among singleton births after blastocyst versus cleavage stage embryo transfer: a systematic review and meta-analysis. *Hum Reprod Update.* 2014;20(3):439–448.

8. Ginstrom Ernstad E, Bergh C, Khatibi A, et al. Neonatal and maternal outcome after blastocyst transfer: a population-based registry study. *Am J Obstet Gynecol.* 2016;214(3):378 e371–378 e310.

9. Fedder J, Loft A, Parner ET, Rasmussen S, Pinborg A. Neonatal outcome and congenital malformations in children born after ICSI with testicular or epididymal sperm: a controlled national cohort study. *Hum Reprod.* 2013;28(1):230–240.

10. Pelkonen S, Hartikainen AL, Ritvanen A, et al. Major congenital anomalies in children born after frozen embryo transfer: a cohort study 1995–2006. *Hum Reprod.* 2014;29(7):1552–1557.

11. *Committee opinion: perinatal risks associated with assisted reproductive technology.* American College of Obstetricians and Gynecologists; 2016.

47

Biomarkers of Ovarian Reserve and Infertility Among Older Reproductive Age Women

ALEXIS GADSON AND WENDY KUOHUNG

"Among late reproductive age women without a history of infertility trying to conceive for 3 months or less, biomarkers indicating diminished ovarian reserve were not associated with reduced fertility."

—AZ STEINER ET AL.[1]

Research Question: Which biomarkers of ovarian reserve are associated with reproductive potential in late reproductive age women?

Funding: National Institute of Health (NHI)/National Institute of Child Health and Human Development R21 and the Intramural Research Program of the NIH, National Institute of Environmental Health Sciences

Year Study Began: 2008

Year Study Published: 2017

Study Location: Raleigh-Durham, North Carolina

Who Was Studied: Women ages 30 to 44 without a history of infertility trying to conceive for 3 months or less and cohabitating with a male partner

Who Was Excluded: History of sterilization, Polycystic Ovarian Syndrome (PCOS), previous or current use of fertility treatments, known tubal blockage, surgically diagnosed endometriosis, partner infertility, breastfeeding, use of injectable hormonal contraception within the last 12 months

Number of Patients: 981

Study Overview: See Figure 47.1

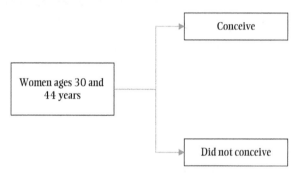

Figure 47.1 Study overview

Women were followed in a prospective, time-to-pregnancy cohort and completed a daily diary, blood anti-Mullerian hormone (AMH), urinary follicle stimulating hormone (FSH), and inhibin B while attempting to conceive. Serum and urine biomarkers were observed for possible correlation between the levels and time to conception.

Follow-Up: Women followed for 6 to 12 months of pregnancy attempt. Women were removed at the initiation of fertility medications, when lost to follow-up, or upon request.

Endpoints: Primary outcome measures for the study were the cumulative probability of conception by 6 menstrual cycles, by 12 menstrual cycles, and relative fecundability. There were no secondary outcomes.

RESULTS

- As women age, AMH levels decrease and FSH increases.
- Obese women have significantly lower AMH and inhibin values.
- The probability of conceiving naturally by 6 cycles or 12 cycles is not lower for women with low AMH or high FSH (see Table 47.1).

- Women without a history of infertility with low AMH values or high serum FSH did not have reduced fecundability.
- Women with high FSH values (>10mIU/ml) did not have a significantly different cumulative probability of conceiving after 6 cycles of naturally attempting pregnancy (see Table 47.1).

Table 47.1. ASSOCIATION BETWEEN BIOMARKERS OF OVARIAN RESERVE AND PREDICTED PROBABILITY OF CONCEIVING

Biomarker	Number	Conceived During Study, Number (%)	Cumulative Probability of Conception[a] (95% CI)		Hazard Ratio (95% CI) Adjusted
			By 6 Cycles	By 12 Cycles	
AMH					
<0.7ng/ml	84	53 (63%)	65% (50,75)	84% (70,91)	1.19 (0.88–1.61)
0.7–8.4mg/ml	579	381 (66%)	62% (57,66)	75% (70,79)	Referent
≥8.5ng/ml	74	44 (59%)	59% (45,69)	66% (57,77)	0.88 (0.64–1.21)
FSH, serum					
<10mIU/ml	654	420 (64%)	62% (57,66)	75% (70,78)	Referent
≥10mIU/ml	83	58 (70%)	63% (50,73)	82% (70,89)	1.22 (0.92–1.62)

[a]Predicted from Cox models adjusted for age, body mass index, race, current smoking status, and recent hormonal contraceptive use.
Abbreviations: CI, confidence interval; AMH, anti-Mullerian hormone; FSH, follicle stimulating hormone.

Criticisms and Limitations: The primary outcome of the study is conception, but the ultimate goal of studies of fecundability should be live birth. The majority of women (69%) enrolled in the study were under the age of 35, the age at which fertility begins to decline, biasing the study toward a positive result. Selection of laboratory cutoff values may have biased study results. The authors selected a serum FSH of 10mIU/ml as the threshold for abnormal, but most clinicians would consider an FSH of 12 to 15mIU to be abnormal. These higher values may more accurately reflect success rates with attempts at conception. Semen samples were not collected for the partners of study participants. While the distribution of partners with abnormal semen analyses theoretically should be evenly spread throughout the study cohort, investigation of age/incidence of abnormal semen analysis in partners may contribute to predicting time to conception.

Not all participants in the study completed the full 12 cycles. Ovulation was not assessed during this study, limiting the ability to evaluate for ovulatory cycles that are crucial to reproductive success. This study was not powered to explore very low AMH values (0.1ng/ml or lower). There may a decrease in fecundability noted at these extremely low levels that is not reflected in the results of this study.

Other Relevant Studies and Information:

- AMH is produced by granulosa cells of developing follicles of the ovary in females and helps control maturation of follicles during the menstrual cycle. Lower AMH means less follicles are available to mature to dominance. This makes AMH a good biomarker for predicting response to ovarian stimulation.[2]
- The American Society for Reproductive Medicine recommends use of multiple assays to assess causes of infertility including measurement of serum AMH. They specifically recommend ovarian reserve testing such as AMH and FSH for women over age 35 years, those with a family history of early menopause, those who have one ovary, those with a history of previous ovarian surgery, those who have undergone chemotherapy or pelvic radiation, and those who are planning treatment with assisted reproductive technology.[3]
- Lower levels of AMH have been associated with poor embryo quality and poor pregnancy outcomes in IVF.[3]

Summary and Implications: Serum biomarkers of diminished ovarian reserve may be a useful tool in counseling infertile patients on their ability to conceive with treatment; however, AMH and FSH levels did not predict fecundability among women without a history of infertility.

CLINICAL CASE

Case History
A 34-year-old gravida 0 single female with a remote history of migraines presents to your clinic desiring fertility preservation. She has never attempted to conceive with a male partner and is interested in egg freezing. She underwent menarche at age 12 and has regular periods that are not heavy. She denies pelvic pain, and she has never used contraception. Her past medical and surgical history are negative, and she is a nonsmoker. You obtain day 3 FSH and AMH for further evaluation. Her results are as follows: serum FSH 15.2mIU/ml, E_2 24, AMH 0.61ng/ml. How will you advise the patient regarding the

likely outcome of oocyte cryopreservation and the likelihood of achieving conception on her own in the future?

Suggested Answer

Based on the results of this study, a provider may counsel this non-infertile patient that abnormal FSH and AMH values do not indicate decreased reproductive potential. A previous study has shown that a combination of age, serum FSH, AMH, and antral follicle count (AFC) provides the most accurate prediction of number of oocytes obtained at retrieval, a corollary of response to ovarian stimulation. Removing serum FSH from the prediction model did not reduce the ability to predict number of oocytes retrieved, but use of age, serum AMH level, and AFC in combination was superior to the use of only one or two variables.[4]

The previous theory that fertility can be predicted based on these biomarkers was not well supported in this cohort of women without a known history of infertility. Ovarian reserve biomarkers can be affected by multiple factors including recent use of hormonal contraceptives and the laboratory assays used for sample analysis. These women should be counseled that while ovarian reserve testing may provide information about overall hormonal status, the AMH and FSH should be one part of a complete evaluation. These values alone may not provide sufficient information regarding future ability to conceive.

References

1. Steiner AZ, Pritchard D, Stanczyk FZ, Kesner JS, Meadows JW, Herring AH, et al. Association between biomarkers of ovarian reserve and infertility among older women of reproductive age. *JAMA.* 2017;318(14):1367–1376. http://jama.jamanetwork.com/article.aspx?doi=10.1001/jama.2017.14588
2. Dewailly D, Andersen CY, Balen A, Broekmans F, Dilaver N, Fanchin R, et al. The physiology and clinical utility of anti-Müllerian hormone in women. *Hum Reprod Update* 2014;20(3):370–385. http://academic.oup.com/humupd/article/20/3/370/731356/The-physiology-and-clinical-utility-of
3. Diagnostic evaluation of the infertile female: a committee opinion. http://dx.doi.org/10.1016/j.fertnstert.2015.03.019
4. Moon KY, Kim H, Lee JY, Lee JR, Jee BC, Suh CS, et al. Nomogram to predict the number of oocytes retrieved in controlled ovarian stimulation. *Clin Exp Reprod Med.* 2016;43(2):112–118. http://synapse.koreamed.org/DOIx.php?id=10.5653/cerm.2016.43.2.112

48

Risks and Benefits of Estrogen Plus Progestin in Healthy Postmenopausal Women

The Women's Health Initiative

RACHEL BEVERLEY AND JUDITH VOLKAR

"This regimen should not be initiated or continued for primary prevention of Coronary Heart Disease."

—WRITING GROUP FOR THE WOMEN'S HEALTH
INITIATIVE INVESTIGATORS[1]

Research Question: What are the health benefits and risks of the most commonly used combined hormone preparation among postmenopausal women in the United States?

Funding: National Heart, Lung, and Blood institute funded the Women's Health Initiative (WHI) program. Wyeth-Ayerst Research provided the study medications.

Year Study Began: 1993

Year Study Published: 2002

Study Location: 40 clinical centers within the United States

Who Was Studied: Postmenopausal women aged 50 to 79 years. Women were considered postmenopausal if they had no vaginal bleeding for 6 months (12 months for women aged 50 to 54), had a prior hysterectomy, or had ever used postmenopausal hormone therapy (HT).

Who Was Excluded: Women with medical conditions with "competing risk," safety concerns, or considered to be at risk for nonadherence or dropout. Such factors included medical conditions associated with a predicted survival of <3 years, history of breast cancer or other prior cancer within 10 years except for nonmelanoma skin cancer, low hematocrit or platelet count, alcoholism, and dementia.

How Many Patients: 16,608

Study Overview: This randomized controlled trial studies hormone therapy for postmenopausal women. See Figure 48.1

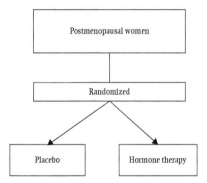

Figure 48.1. Study overview: the Women's Health Initiative

Study Intervention: Patients in the combined estrogen and progestin (E+P) group received 1 daily tablet containing conjugated equine estrogen (CEE) 0.625mg and medroxyprogesterone acetate (MPA) 2.5mg. Patients in the placebo group took a placebo tablet once daily.

Follow-Up: Participants had telephone follow-up 6 weeks after randomization. Additional follow-up occurred every 6 months with annual clinic visits required. The trial was planned to have 8.5 years of follow-up.

Endpoints: Primary outcome: Coronary heart disease (CHD) (nonfatal myocardial infarction and CHD death). Primary adverse outcome: Invasive breast cancer. A global index was used to summarize the balance of risks and benefits and included CHD, invasive breast cancer, stroke, pulmonary embolism, endometrial cancer, colorectal cancer, hip fracture, and death due to other causes.

RESULTS

- The study ended early after the 10th interim analysis (2002) due to concern for increased risk of breast cancer; the global index was supportive of a finding of overall harm.
- Baseline characteristics for groups were similar (mean age 63.3±7.1 years).
- In the E+P arm relative to placebo:
  - The rate of CHD events was increased by 29% (7 additional events per 10,000 person-years [py]).
  - The rate of stroke was increased by 41% (8/10,000py).
  - The rate of invasive breast cancer was increased by 26% (8/10,000py).
  - There was a 2-fold greater rate of venous thromboembolism (VTE) (18/10,000py).
  - The rate of colorectal cancer was reduced by 37% (6 fewer colon cancers per 10,000py). See Table 48.1.

Table 48.1. SUMMARY OF STUDY'S KEY FINDINGS

	No. of Patients (Annualized %)		Hazard Ratio	Nominal 95% CI
	Estrogen+Progestin (*n* = 8,506)	Placebo (*n* = 8,102)		
Total CVD	694 (1.57)	546 (1.32)	1.22	1.09–1.36
Invasive breast cancer	166 (0.38)	124 (0.30)	1.26	1.00–1.59
Colorectal cancer	45 (0.10)	67 (0.16)	0.63	0.43–0.92
Total fractures	650 (1.47)	788 (1.91)	0.76	0.69–0.85
Global index[a]	751 (1.70)	623 (1.51)	1.15	1.03–1.28

[a]Global index included CHD, stroke, pulmonary embolism, breast cancer, endometrial cancer, colorectal cancer, hip fracture, and death due to other causes.
Abbreviations: CI, confidence interval; CVD, cardiovascular disease.

Criticisms and Limitations: The WHI trial tested only one HT regimen—an oral regimen with fixed doses of CEE and MPA. Additionally, there was limited enrollment of women <60 years old and <10 years from menopause with bothersome vasomotor symptoms—the patient population that would likely benefit most from HT. Results are difficult to generalize to current practice given use of different forms and dosages of E+P and available routes of administration. The trial did not include any analysis by age of participants or years since menopause. Interpretation of the WHI data should be viewed with caution—the relative risks are increased for various outcomes outlined here; however, the absolute increase in these events was quite small.

Other Relevant Studies and Information:

- The WHI has published multiple studies examining potential risks and benefits of HT in postmenopausal women. Secondary analyses have found that women who initiate HT closer to menopause have a trend toward reduced CHD risk compared to women who initiated HT more distant from menopause.[2]
- The position statement from the North American Menopause Society states that women <60 years old who are within 10 years of menopause have the most favorable benefit-risk ratio for use of HT to treat bothersome vasomotor symptoms.[3] Multiple smaller studies have also demonstrated an improved safety profile of transdermal formulations in regards to VTE risk.

Summary and Implications: The authors of the WHI concluded that risks of HT, including breast cancer and cardiovascular disease, outweighed the benefits of therapy including a reduction of fractures. However, because these risks are relatively small, it appears to be appropriate to initiate HT for women with bothersome vasomotor symptoms who are within 10 years of the onset of menopause and are healthy, especially once other therapies have been shown to be ineffective.

CLINICAL CASE: RISKS AND BENEFITS OF ESTROGEN PLUS PROGESTIN IN HEALTHY POSTMENOPAUSAL WOMEN

Case History

A healthy 53-year-old woman presents to your office with complaints of hot flashes, night sweats, and vaginal dryness for 18 months. She reports absence of menses for 13 months. She is interested in initiating HT but expresses concern regarding safety. How would you counsel her regarding the risks and benefits of systemic HT for her bothersome vasomotor symptoms?

Suggested Answer

This patient is healthy without contraindications to HT. She has a uterus, so E+P therapy is recommended. You counsel her that overall risks of E+P HT (based on initial results of the WHI from 2002) include a small elevation in risk of CHD, myocardial infarction, stroke, VTE, and breast cancer. Benefits include a small decrease in colorectal cancer and fracture risk. Her risk of VTE can be decreased with use of transdermal estrogen preparations. Given that she is <10 years from menopause, more recent data suggests there is not increased CHD risk with use of HT. Her risk of invasive breast cancer will increase as her duration of usage increases, but absolute risk is low. After discussion with the patient regarding HT risks as well as nonhormonal options for symptom management, she makes an informed decision to proceed with therapy. Her individual risk and benefits will be discussed at future visits and managed as they change over time.

References

1. Writing Group for the Women's Health Initiative Investigators. Risks and benefits of estrogen plus progestin and healthy postmenopausal women: principal results from the Women's Health Initiative randomized controlled trial. *JAMA.* 2002 Jul 17;288(3):321–333.
2. Rossouw JE, Prentice RL, Manson JE, et al. Postmenopausal hormone therapy and risk of cardiovascular disease by age and year since menopause. *JAMA.* 2007 Apr 4;297 (13):1465–1477.
3. The 2017 hormone therapy position statement of the North American Menopause Society. *Menopause.* 2017;24(7):728–753.

Predictors of Success of Methotrexate Treatment for Tubal Ectopic Pregnancies

MARY LOUISE FOWLER, PAUL HENDESSI, AND NYIA NOEL

"Many women with ectopic pregnancies are now treated with methotrexate instead of surgery [. . .] but it has been difficult to determine the true effect of [characteristics affecting success with methotrexate] because of the small size of previous studies."

—GH LIPSCOMB ET AL.[1]

Research Question: What pretreatment factors, if any, play a role in the success of single-dose methotrexate protocol in women with tubal ectopic pregnancies?

Funding: Not reported

Year Study Began: Not reported

Year Study Published: 1999

Study Location: Memphis, Tennessee

Who Was Studied: Women with singleton tubal ectopic pregnancies who were hemodynamically stable and willing to participate in treatment with intramuscular (IM) methotrexate (MTX). Inclusion criteria required the size of the gestational mass to be 3.5cm or less, or up to 4.0cm if no fetal cardiac activity was present.

Who Was Excluded: Women who were hemodynamically unstable, had free fluid (presumably blood) outside of the pelvic cavity as demonstrated on transvaginal ultrasound (TVUS), had non-tubal ectopic pregnancies, did not agree to weekly follow-up, or elected to have surgical rather than medical management. Women were also excluded if they had hepatic, hematologic, or renal disease.

How Many Patients: 350

Study Overview: See Figure 49.1

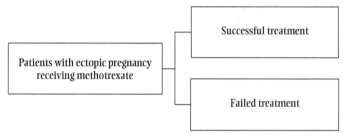

Figure 49.1. Study overview

Study Intervention: Women with tubal ectopic pregnancies were treated with IM MTX according to a single dose protocol, with repeat administrations per protocol if hCG did not decrease appropriately or with continued fetal cardiac activity. Treatment was deemed a failure if surgical management was indicated or after 3 doses of MTX without resolution of the ectopic pregnancy. An exception was made in 1 case where 4 doses of MTX were allowed.

Follow-Up: Women were followed until resolution of their ectopic pregnancy, either by surgical management or with hCG reaching a value of 15mIU/mL or less.

Endpoints: The primary outcome was successful treatment of ectopic pregnancy via MTX management.

RESULTS

- Among 350 women, 320 (91%) were successfully treated and 261 (82%) only required 1 dose.
- Serum progesterone concentration and presence of fetal cardiac activity were higher in women requiring more than one dose of MTX ($p < 0.001$).

- There was no relationship between age, parity, size or volume of conceptus, or presence of fluid in peritoneal cavity and efficacy of treatment.
- Fetal cardiac activity was initially present in 12% of successfully treated cases and 30% of those in which treatment was unsuccessful ($p = 0.01$).
- Regression analysis revealed pretreatment hCG to be the only factor that contributed to the failure rate. See Table 49.1.

Table 49.1. ANALYSIS OF FACTORS RELATED TO THE EFFICACY OF METHOTREXATE THERAPY IN WOMEN WITH ECTOPIC PREGNANCIES

Factor	Success ($n = 320$)	Failure ($n = 30$)	p-value
Serum hCG (mIU/mL)	4019+/− 6362	13420+/− 16590	<0.001
Serum progesterone (ng/mL)	6.9+/−6.7	10.2+/− 5.5	0.02
Presence of fetal cardiac activity, number (%)	37 (12%)	9 (30%)	0.01

Age, parity, size of mass, and presence of free peritoneal fluid were not predictors of outcome

---

Criticisms and Limitations: The trial did not mention the follow-up adherence of patients, and it appears they had perfect follow-up, which is not always practical or reproducible. The length of follow-up required to reach a level of 15mIU/mL was not discussed. In addition, the socioeconomic status of the patients is not known. In one study, patients with low socioeconomic status were 5 times as likely to fail MTX treatment.[2] The study also presumed that at an hCG of 2000mIU/mL, one should be able to identify an intrauterine pregnancy (IUP) on TVUS. The study states that an increase in hCG at this point when no IUP is visualized signifies an ectopic pregnancy. However, it is possible that these patients had an IUP that was too early to visualize on TVUS. The value of hCG should be conservatively high (i.e. 3,500 mIU/mL) to avoid the potential for misdiagnosing an IUP as an ectopic.[3] This may have also led to falsely elevated success rates of MTX management. Finally, this study does not provide long-term follow-up of time to future pregnancy.

Other Relevant Studies and Information:

- Some 2-dose and multidose protocols have demonstrated greater levels of success than single-dose protocols, particularly in atypical ectopic pregnancies, including cesarean scar ectopic[4] and patients with higher initial hCG levels.[5,6]

- A study by Mergenthal et al. of 162 racially and geographically diverse group of women found that the single- and 2-dose protocols had similar outcomes. The rates of treatment success were comparable (84% for single-dose vs. 79% for 2-dose, $p = .53$) with no significant difference in time to resolution (hazards ratio 0.441; 95% confidence interval 0.139–1.401; $p = .165$).[7]
- A systematic review also showed a failure rate of 14.3% or higher with MTX when pretreatment hCG levels >5,000 compared with 3.7% failure rate for hCG levels <5,000.[8]
- The use of MTX necessitates multiple office visits and surveillance of hCG values for weeks. One study assessing compliance of MTX therapy noted that only 45.5% of patients completed follow-up—and only 19.7% completed "appropriate" follow-up, which was defined as returning day 4, day 7, and weekly until serum hCG levels reached zero.[9] A total of 24% of patients in this group required surgery.
- Currently American College of Obstetricians and Gynecologists guidelines recommend a single-dose methotrexate strategy for most patients, with consideration of a 2-dose protocol for some patients, including those with initial high hCG levels.[10]

Summary and Implications: Among women with tubal ectopic pregnancies, increased hCG, progesterone levels, and cardiac activity are associated with increased failure rates of MTX. The size of the ectopic pregnancy and presence of free peritoneal blood were not associated with failure rate. The predictive factors noted earlier, coupled with the life circumstances and patient preference, may help guide the decision between treatment with MTX versus laparoscopic surgery.

CLINICAL CASE

Case History

A 30-year-old G1P0 with LMP 6 weeks ago presents to the emergency department with vaginal spotting and cramping and a serum hCG of 2700. A TVUS demonstrates no IUP but a 2cm echogenic mass in the right adnexa with cardiac activity. Her vitals are stable. This is a desired pregnancy. She is requesting to not have surgery. How would you counsel this patient?

Suggested Answer

This study demonstrated that for women with tubal ectopic pregnancies, the most important factor associated with failure of treatment with a single-dose methotrexate protocol was a high serum hCG. This case demonstrates a patient with an unruptured ectopic pregnancy and, in particular, is a patient who would be a good candidate for medical management. She is hemodynamically stable, requesting a nonsurgical option. Important factors to consider are her ability to follow up for repeat blood tests, ensuring that the patient has no absolute contraindications to MTX, including hematologic, hepatic, and renal disease. The patient should also be counseled that if her serum hCG does not adequately decrease despite several doses of methotrexate, she might ultimately require surgery.

References

1. Lipscomb GH, McCord ML, Stovall TG, Huff G, Portera SG, Ling FW. Predictors of success of methotrexate treatment in women with tubal ectopic pregnancies. *N Engl J Med.* 1999;341(26);1974–1981.
2. Butts SF, Gibson E, Sammel MD, Shaunik A, Rudick B, Barnhart K. Race, socioeconomic status and response to methotrexate treatment of ectopic pregnancy in an urban population. *Fertil Steril.* 2010 Dec; 94(7):2789–2792.
3. Doubilet PM, Benson CB, Bourne T, Blaivas M, Barnhart KT, Benacerraf BR, et al. Diagnostic criteria for nonviable pregnancy early in the first trimester. Society of Radiologists in Ultrasound Multispecialty Panel on Early First Trimester Diagnosis of Miscarriage and Exclusion of a Viable Intrauterine Pregnancy. *N Engl J Med.* 2013;369:1443–1451.
4. Kutuk MS, Uysal G, Dolanbay M, Ozgun MT. Successful medical treatment of cesarean scar ectopic pregnancies with systemic multidose methotrexate: single-center experience. *J Obstet Gynacol Res.* 2014 Jun; 40(6): 1700–1706.
5. Hamed HO, Ahmed SR, Alghasham AA. Comparison of double- and single-dose methotrexate protocols for treatment of ectopic pregnancy. *Int J Gynaecol Obstet.* 2012;116:67–71.
6. Yang C, Cai J, Geng Y, Gao Y. Multiple-dose and double-dose versus single-dose administration of methotrexate for the treatment of ectopic pregnancy: a systematic review and meta-analysis. *Reprod Biomed Online.* 2017;34:383–391.
7. Mergenthal MC, Senapati S, Zee J, Allen-Taylor L, Whittaker PG, Takacs P, Sammel MD, Barnhart KT. Medical management of ectopic pregnancy with single-dose and 2-dose methotrexate protocols: human chorionic gonadotropin trends and patient outcomes. *Am J Obstet Gynecol.* 2016; 215:590.e1–5.
8. Menon S, Colins J, Barnhart KT. Establishing a human chorionic gonadotropin cutoff to guide methotrexate treatment of ectopic pregnancy: a systematic review. *Fertil Steril.* 2007;87:481–484.
9. Jaspan D, Giraldo-Isaza M, Dandolu V, Cohen AW. Compliance with methotrexate therapy for presumed ectopic pregnancy in an inner-city population. *Fertil Steril.* 2010;94:1122–1124.
10. ACOG Practice Bulletin No. 193: tubal ectopic pregnancy: correction. *Obstet Gynecol.* 2019 May;133(5):1059. doi:10.1097/AOG.0000000000003269. PubMed PMID: 31022116

Application of Redefined Human Chorionic Gonadotropin Curves for the Diagnosis of Women at Risk for Ectopic Pregnancy

PAUL TYAN AND LAUREN D. SCHIFF

"[U]se of these new rules will optimize the care of women with an undiagnosed symptomatic first-trimester pregnancy."

—BE SEEBER ET AL.[1]

Research Question: Does application of redefined human chorionic gonadotropin (hCG) diagnostic criteria improve accuracy and time-to-diagnosis of an ectopic pregnancy?

Funding: National Institutes of Health.

Study Years: January 1990 through July 1999

Publication Year: 2006

Study Location: University of Pennsylvania Medical Center, Philadelphia, Pennsylvania

Who Was Studied: Women who presented to the emergency department (ED) with symptoms related to a first-trimester pregnancy and without a definitive diagnosis of intrauterine or extrauterine pregnancy at that initial visit. Women were retrospectively included in this historical cohort study, if they had at least

2 hCG levels collected 24 hours or more apart and a definitive final diagnosis of either an intrauterine pregnancy (IUP), spontaneous abortion (SAB), or ectopic pregnancy (EP).

Who Was Excluded: None

How Many Patients: 124

Study Overview: See Figure 50.1

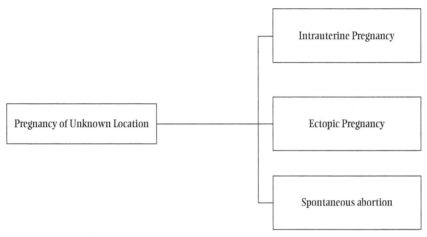

Figure 50.1. Study overview

Study Intervention: The authors applied serial hCG trends from a prior study.[2] A varied lower bound of hCG rise over 2 days for ultimately normal IUP (at the 99.9% confidence interval [CI] 35%) and upper bound of fall of hCG over 2 days for diagnosed SAB were applied to a historical cohort to predict a final diagnosis of either an EP, IUP, or SAB. Different confidence intervals of these bounds of hCG rise and fall were tested in combination to evaluate the performance in predicting diagnosis and minimization of error. Authors also tested a model that used 3 data hCG points over 4 days in determining the diagnosis. The authors prioritized interruption of a normal IUP as the most unfavorable error, followed by failure to identify an EP, and then unnecessary intervention in an SAB.

Follow-Up: Not applicable

Endpoints: Primary outcome: Accuracy and time-to-diagnosis using several different confidence intervals were compared to identify the model that had the least composite potential for error as defined by the authors.

RESULTS

- A model applying a lower bound of 99.9% CI of hCG rise for an IUP (correlating to a 35% increase over 24 to 48 hours) and the upper bound of 90% CI fall in hCG for an SAB (correlating to a 21% to 35% fall over 24 to 48 hours) yielded what the authors determined is the optimal balance between accuracy and time reduction in diagnosis.
- The sensitivity for EP using the diagnostic rule in this optimized model was 83%. Specificity was 95%.
- A model using the same upper and lower bounds of CI did have improved specificity (meaning fewer misclassifications of IUP or SAB) but at the expense of a higher rate of missed EP and longer time-to-diagnosis of EP (1.59 days vs. 2.64 days saved when compared to standard clinical practice).
- The model with the highest sensitivity for EP would have missed fewer EP compared with the optimal model (9.2% vs. 17.3%) but would have potentially resulted in a much higher rate of interrupted IUP (22.2% vs. 4.6%).
- With the application of the new diagnostic rule of a minimum of 35% rise and 21% to 35% fall of 2 consecutive hCG values, the diagnosis of an EP is made 2.5 days sooner than standard clinical practice in the cohort being evaluated.

Table 50.1. SUMMARY OF KEY FINDINGS

Values Based on the Different CI for the Rise of hCG in an IUP and the Fall of hCG in an SAB (1, 2)

Model Type	Optimal Model Recommended by the Authors[a]	Model with the Highest Sensitivity	Model with the Highest Specificity[b]
IUP (CI percentile), **SAB** (CI percentile)	IUP (0.999), SAB (0.90)[a]	IUP (0.95), SAB (0.90)	IUP (0.999), SAB (0.90)[b]
Sensitivity (%)	83	91	79
Specificity (%)	95	78	98
Mean of Days Saved (Range)	2.64 (0–34)	2.94 (0–34)	1.59 (0–34)
Mean of Visits Saved (Range)	1.22 (0–9)	1.35 (0–9)	0.72 (0–9)
Number of Missed EPs (%)	34 (17.3)	18 (9.2)	41 (20.9)
Number of Interrupted IUPs (%)	12 (4.6)	58 (22.2)	6 (2.2)
Number of Unnecessary Intervention for SABs (%)	222 (28.0)	225 (28.4)	189 (23.9)

[a]Minimal rise of 35% in 2 days and minimal fall of 21% to 35%. [b] Over 3 values. Abbreviations: CI, confidence interval; hCG, human chorionic gonadotropin; IUP, intrauterine pregnancy; SAB, spontaneous abortion; EP, ectopic pregnancy.

- Review of ultrasounds suggested that all 12 patients with an eventual IUP that might have been misdiagnosed as an EP by the optimal model criteria had ultrasound findings suggestive of an early IUP. See Table 50.1.

Criticisms and Limitations:

- Even though the suggested model improves on time-to-diagnosis, there is still a small risk of interrupting a potentially viable pregnancy. As the authors themselves emphasize, interventions should not be undertaken based solely on hCG rise or fall but should take into account the clinical picture, patient preferences, and other data including ultrasound.
- The hCG trends used to apply the suggested curves were derived from the same patient population used to build the initial curves; these curves may potentially not be generalizable to other populations.

Other Relevant Studies and Information:

- hCG levels trend should not be used solely to diagnose an EP. A complete assessment of gestational age, ultrasound findings, and clinical exam should build the framework that ultimately drives the management plan.[3,4]
- A subsequent study found that hCG levels increase in a curvilinear fashion; the expected rate off rise can be as low as 33% if the initial hCG is greater than 3000mIU/mL. Thus, hCG trends must take into account the initial hCG level.[5]
- Further studies have resulted in the modification of guidelines for the ultrasound criteria used to diagnose IUP and pregnancy failure. These include changed criteria for the discriminatory zone at which IUP should first be visualized on ultrasound (hCG level of ß 3500 rather than a previously defined discriminatory zone of 1500 to 2000)[6,7] and more conservative ultrasound criteria for the diagnosis of pregnancy failure, including a crown-rump length of ≥7 mm with no heartbeat and a mean sac diameter of ≥25mm with no embryo.[7]
- Endometrial sampling for aid in diagnosing a Pregnancy of Unknown Location (PUL) in patients presenting with undesired pregnancy remains an essential tool for diagnosis and treatment.[8]
- American College of Obstetricians and Gynecologists (ACOG) guidelines currently recommend using a minimum 33% rise in hCG to predict possible IUP and a minimum decrease of 21% to 36% to predict possible SAB.[9]

Summary and Implications: This analysis identified a framework to assess hCG trends in early pregnancy to diagnose an EP while keeping a low risk to interrupt an IUP and to prevent unnecessary diagnostic procedures in women with SAB who present with symptoms concerning for possible EP. Based on this study and others, ACOG guidelines recommend management of early pregnancy of unknown location based on the metrics of this study and emphasizes the recommendations based on patient-guided decision-making.

CLINICAL CASE

Case History

A clinically stable 28-year-old G2P0010 presents to the ED complaining of lower pelvic pain and spotting for 24 hours. She had a positive home pregnancy test with a last menstrual period 5 weeks prior. In the ED, her hCG was 1080mIU/mL, and the transvaginal ultrasound showed a gestational sac of 7mm and no yolk sac. The patient had normal vitals and a nonperitoneal abdomen on exam. A repeat hCG in 48 hours detected a 32% increase from her baseline hCG. What is the next best step in management?

Suggested Answer

This patient presents with symptoms that are concerning for possible EP. Her ultrasound is not diagnostic, and her hCG rise is slightly less than the 33% increase in hCG at 24 to 48 hours that is at the 99.9% CI of rise that predicts a normal pregnancy. Subsequent interventions such as uterine aspiration or close follow-up should be achieved through shared decision-making after thorough counseling backed by objective evidence. The patient should be counseled regarding the lower likelihood of IUP but should also be counseled that dilation and curettage does include a small risk of interruption of a viable IUP. Continued expectant management with serial hCG and ultrasound is a reasonable approach to care as long as the patient is stable, is well-counseled regarding the risk and possible consequences of ruptured ectopic, is given strict symptom precautions for recognition of possible ruptured ectopic, and desires this type of management.

References

1. Seeber BE, Sammel MD, Guo W, Zhou L, Hummel A, Barnhart KT. Application of redefined human chorionic gonadotropin curves for the diagnosis of women at risk for ectopic pregnancy. *Fertil Steril.* 2006;86(2):454–459.

2. Barnhart K, Sammel MD, Chung K, Zhou L, Hummel AC, Guo W. Decline of serum human chorionic gonadotropin and spontaneous complete abortion: defining the normal curve. *Obstet Gynecol.* 2004;104:975–981.

3. Seeber BE. What serial hCG can tell you, and cannot tell you, about an early pregnancy. *Fertil Steril.* 2012;98(5):1074.

4. Morse CB, Sammel MD, Shaunik A, Allen-Taylor L, Oberfoell NL, Takacs P, et al. Performance of human chorionic gonadotropin curves in women at risk for ectopic pregnancy: exceptions to the rules. *Fertil Steril.* 2012;97:101–106.e2.

5. Barnhart KT, Guo W, Cary MS, Morse CB, Chung K, Takacs P, et al. Differences in serum human chorionic gonadotropin rise in early pregnancy by race and value at presentation. *Obstet Gynecol.* 2016;128:504–511.

6. Connolly A, Ryan DH, Stuebe AM, Wolfe HM. Reevaluation of discriminatory and threshold levels for serum beta-hCG in early pregnancy. *Obstet Gynecol.* 2013;121:65–70.

7. Doubilet PM, Benson CB, Bourne T, Blaivas M, Barnhart KT, Benacerraf BR, et al. Diagnostic criteria for nonviable pregnancy early in the first trimester. Society of Radiologists in Ultrasound Multispecialty Panel on Early First Trimester Diagnosis of Miscarriage and Exclusion of a Viable Intrauterine Pregnancy. *N Engl J Med.* 2013; 369:1443–1451.

8. Shaunik A, Kulp J, Appleby DH, Sammel MD, Barnhart KT. Utility of dilation and curettage in the diagnosis of pregnancy of unknown location. *AJOG.* 2011;204:130e1–6.

9. ACOG Practice Bulletin No. 193: tubal ectopic pregnancy: correction. *Obstet Gynecol.* 2019 May;133(5):1059. doi:10.1097/AOG.0000000000003269. PubMed PMID: 31022116

INDEX

Tables, figures and boxes are indicated by *t, f* and *b* following the page number

CPSIA information can be obtained
at www.ICGtesting.com
Printed in the USA
BVHW052028250623
666323BV00001B/2